This book is jointly published by Times Editions Pte Ltd,
Eu Yan Sang Holdings Ltd and CRCS Publications

Cover photography by Lawrence Lim

Photographs on pages 2, 4, 6, 41–43, 73–75 and 115–117 by
Lawrence Lim. All photographs of plants and herbs by Wee Yeow
Chin except *Acanthopanax gracilistylus* (p. 15), *Citrus aurantium*
(p. 58), *Euonymus alata* (p. 81), *Ginkgo biloba* (p. 90), *Glycyrrhiza
glabra* (p. 91), *Juglans regia* (p. 102), *Phyllostachys nigra* (p. 135),
Pyrrosia lingua (p. 153), *Rhus verniciflua* (p. 158), *Ziziphus jujuba*
(p. 179) and *Rubus parvifolius* (p. 161) by Prof Lee Kavaljian of
California State University, Sacramento; and *Angelica* (p. 26),
Bambusa (p. 38), *Paeonia suffruticosa* (p. 87) and *Viola chinensis*
(p. 175) by Gertrude Looi.

The publishers wish to thank Mrs Gertrude Looi for initiating the
production of this book and for her considerable
contribution to it in more ways than one.

North American Edition © 1992 CRCS Publications
Original edition © 1990 Times Editions Pte Ltd
Times Centre
1 New Industrial Road
Singapore 1953

FOR SALE IN THE USA AND CANADA ONLY

Library of Congress Cataloguing-in-Publication Data
Wee, Yeow Chin.
    An illustrated dictionary of Chinese medicinal herbs.
        p.   cm.
    Authors: Wee Yeow Chin and Hsuan Keng.
    Includes indexes.
    ISBN 0-916360-53-9 : $32.95
    1. Herbs—China—Therapeutic use—Dictionaries.   2. Materia
medica, Vegetable—China—Dictionaries.   3. Medicinal plants—
China—Dictionaries.   I. Keng, Hsuan, 1923–   II. Title.
RM666.H33W38   1992
615' .321 ' 0951—dc20
                                                                  91–40789
                                                                       CIP

Set in Garamond, 11 points over 13 points
Printed in Singapore by Kyodo Printing Co (S'pore) Pte Ltd

ISBN 0-916360-53-9

An Illustrated Dictionary of

CHINESE MEDICINAL HERBS

Wee Yeow Chin & Hsuan Keng

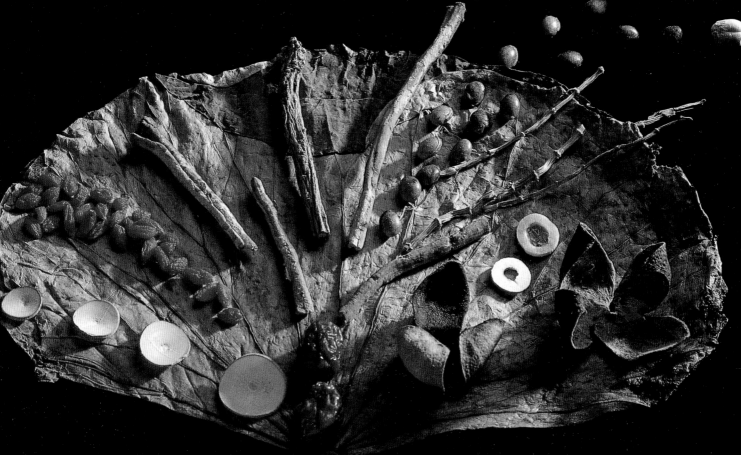

CRCS PUBLICATIONS

Post Office Box 1460
Sebastopol, California 95472

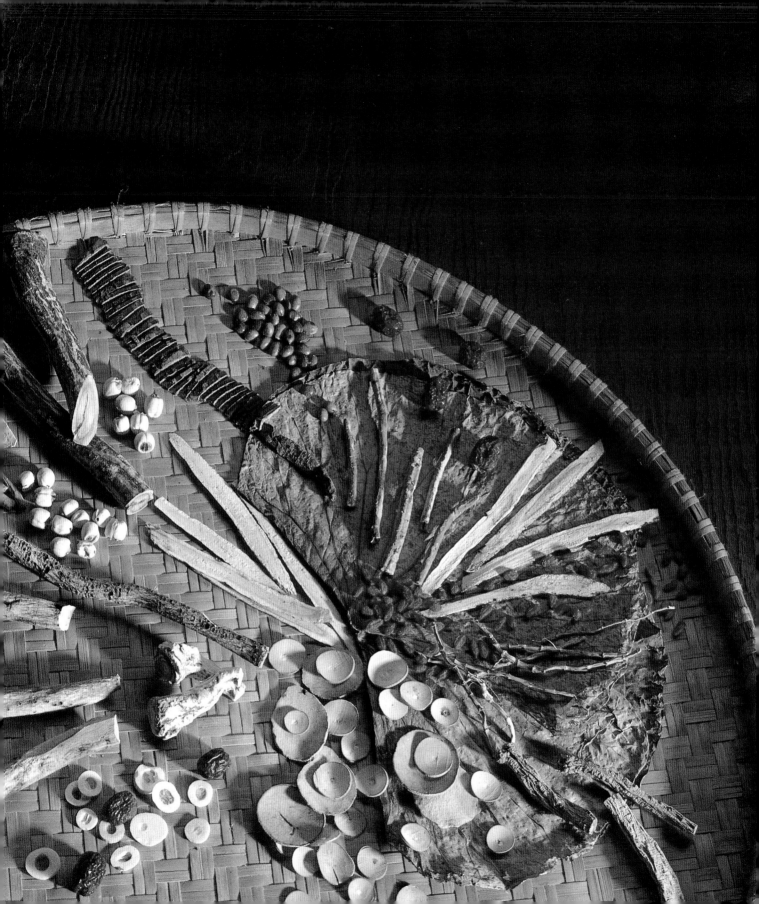

Contents

Opposite page: Herbs are seldom imbibed singly but are combined for the best effect; sometimes one herb balances another to reduce potency, or increases the effect. Ji zi (Lycium chinense) is added to the heating dang gui (Angelica sinensis) to make it less yang, red dates added to dang gui makes it more yang. Several herbal brews have multiple effects and are taken as tonics simply to aid normal body functions or for general debility, e.g. eight pearls soup and bak kut teh.

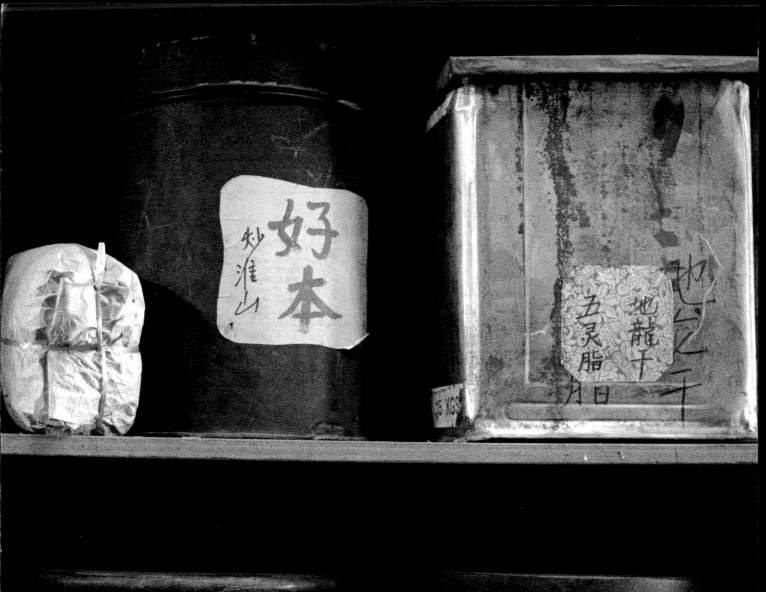
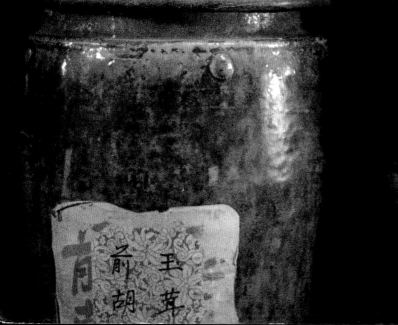
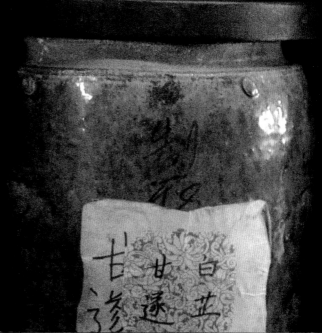

are used to
herbs that are
d in solutions.

Foreword

Nature has always been the Great Provider. Throughout human history, Man has sought sustenance and shelter and, without fail, found them in Nature's realm. And so it was that over time, Man began to use the open laboratory that is the earth to seek cures for common ailments and more complex diseases. Nature has also become the Great Healer. From the time of the almost mystical panaceas offered by the ancient Egyptians to the recent surge of interest in "nature medicine", the significance of this early branch of the medicine tree cannot be overlooked.

For more than 4000 years, the Chinese have been developing and refining medicinal treatments based on the raw ingredients of plants. Over a billion people now subscribe to the natural healing powers of herbs and their derivatives.

Practitioners of Chinese medicine respond to individual complaints and recommend a prescription based on the established traditions of *yin* and *yang*. In Singapore and Malaysia, one of the oldest and most respected of this special breed of practitioners is the Eu Yan Sang chain of medicine shops. In the mid-1870s Eu Kong left his village in southern China to seek his fortune in what was then known as Malaya. He took with him a collection of Chinese herbs and generations of accumulated knowledge.

Eu Kong started the first Eu Yan Sang shop in 1879, dispensing medicines based on both local and imported ingredients. The expertise of the shop's Chinese herbalists and the high quality of their prescriptions ensured the success of the shop. The business was then expanded by his entrepreneurial son, Eu Tong Sen. Today a network of Eu Yan Sang stores bear the legacy of the fine tradition began by Eu Kong.

This book takes a Western approach in the hope of removing some of the mystery surrounding Chinese medicine and explains, in Western terms, the various natural ingredients to be found in Chinese medicine shops. The result, we hope, is a better understanding of an age-old tradition, and an even greater appreciation of the wonders of nature.

Richard Keng Mun Eu
Chairman
Eu Yan Sang Holdings Ltd
September 1990

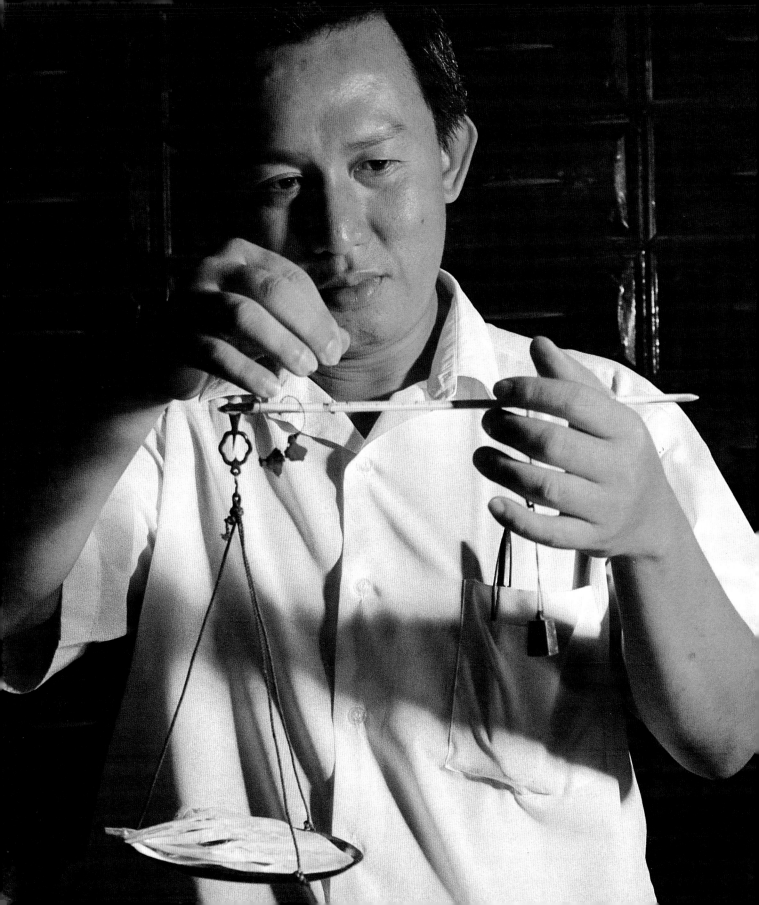

INTRODUCTION

In the present day of western influence through education, the media and ease of travel, the younger generations of ethnic Chinese are led to believe that Chinese medicine is outdated and that to partake in it is not the "in" thing, if not outright old fashioned. But then, is this totally true? Are Chinese medicinal herbs all that useless, as some may claim? Are all traditional medicines to be discarded outright?

Traditional Chinese medicine did not develop overnight – it has a very long history. However, contrary to general belief, it is not the world's earliest recorded medical system. The Egyptians and the Babylonians predated the Chinese in this field by at least a thousand years. However, Chinese medicine is the oldest continuous surviving tradition, rivalled only by Ayurvedic (literally, the "knowledge of longevity") medicine in India.

Chinese medicine has always been associated with three legendary emperors: Fu Si (伏羲), Shen Nong (神农) and Huang Di (黄帝). Fu Si, whose reign was said to have started in 2852 B.C., has been credited with the authorship of the classic, *Yi Jing* (易经) or *Book of Changes*, which laid down the *yin-yang* doctrine. The second legendary emperor, Shen Nong, or the god of husbandry, is reputed to be the earliest Chinese herbalist. To him is attributed the authorship of the first herbal classic, *Shen Nong's Herbal Classic* (神农本草经). Shen Nong (3737–2697 B.C.) was said to have personally tasted many of the herbs, including numerous poisonous ones. The third emperor, Huang Di (2697–2595 B.C.), or Yellow Emperor, is credited with the authorship of *Huang Di Nei Jing* (黄帝内经), or the *Yellow Emperor's Inner Classic*. This classic is the first complete summary of ancient Chinese medicine and is a complete treatise on the principles of health and medicine.

Most scholars of Chinese medicine accept its legendary origin in faith. However, it is probable

7

that knowledge of herbal medicine evolved through the centuries as a result of man's trials and errors in his dealings with the world around him. It can safely be assumed that knowledge of Chinese herbs originated from the earliest inhabitants in China. As they became familiar with the plants around them, seeking out the edible ones, they were bound to come across the disagreeable as well as the agreeable. They were also bound to experience various reactions in their attempts at consuming the plants: from mild to violent reactions, depending on how poisonous the plants were. In the process, they would gradually become familiar with the poisonous plants and those that could relieve pain and illness. And, through the years, such knowledge of the healing properties of plants would naturally accumulate.

Superstitions also contributed to the use of plants for medicinal purposes. The ancients believed that plants somehow developed specific appearances to indicate their curative properties. Thus a decoction of the thorns of *Gleditsia* or *Ziziphus* was used to accelerate the bursting of abscesses, the yellow bark of *Berberis* for jaundice, the red root of *Rubia cordifolia* to increase menstrual flow, the faeces of bats to treat night blindness, and the moulted skins of snakes for skin problems. The most well known of Chinese herbs, the ginseng, with its branching roots which resemble the human figure, appears to be a panacea for nearly all human ills.

This belief was not confined to the Chinese. The Greek philosopher, Theophratus, reported that the root of the polypody fern, rough and with suckers like the tentacles of a polyp, would prevent a person from getting rectal polyps if he wore it as an amulet. Herbalists in Egypt and ancient Babylon made use of the lungs of a fox for the treatment of chronic respiratory problems and cashew nuts for kidney problems. The American Indians eliminated worms by eating a wormlike plant part such as the tendrils of a squash; to promote lactation they used a plant with a milky sap, and a piece of gnarled wood was placed next to a convulsive person. In Southeast Asia, the pencil tree, or milkbush (*Euphorbia tirucalli*), a cactus-like tree with thin branches that resemble bones (hence the Malay name, *tulang tulang*, or "bones"), is prescribed for painful bones and joints. The Javanese use the white, poisonous latex from the branches of the tree to heal fractured bones.

It was the Swiss alchemist and physician Paracelsus (1490–1541) who developed this idea further, naming it the doctrine of signatures. According to this doctrine, diseases were thought to be manifestations of the devil, thus their cures were made available by God in the form of plants. The signs or "signatures" are usually the appearance of the whole plant or its various parts, be it its shape or colour. Thus the kidney bean, with its kidney-like appearance, would naturally cure urinary afflictions, while the walnut, which looks like a human brain, would cure madness or even migraine headaches. By the same token, the Dutchman's Pipe (*Aristolochia*), with its flowers looking like a womb, was thought to be useful in difficult births. Plants possessing a yellow latex were believed to affect the bile, while red beetroot was good for the blood and red wines were used for the treatment of anaemia.

Traditional Chinese medicine was also exposed to foreign influence, although much later, through trade, especially by India's Ayurvedic medicine which reached China around 300 to 200 B.C. Medicinal herbs from India subsequently found their way into China, as can be seen from the listing in a number of early Chinese books on medicinal herbs.

Before the advent of the written language, knowledge of medicinal herbs was passed on from one generation to the next by word of mouth. However, once written language was evolved, records could be made and prescriptions appeared. Archaeological evidence shows that the earliest Chinese characters, which appeared as far back as 3000 years ago, were inscribed on tortoise shells and ox bones; many of these characters are about human illnesses. Later, records were carved on stone, the earliest of which were the Dragon Gate Prescriptions, done some 1400 years ago and found in a cave in Henan Province. There were about 100 prescriptions, remedies for a variety of ailments.

With the availability of paper, record keeping became simpler. The earliest book containing information on Chinese herbs is the *Shi Jing*（诗经）, or the *Book of Poetry*, which includes much information on the gathering of herbs. Compiled during the period 770 to 746 B.C., this classic is said to have been edited by Confucius himself. The first complete summary of ancient Chinese medicine, *Huang Di Nei Jing*, or *Yellow Emperor's Inner Classic*, was probably written by medical scholars during the Warring States Period (475–221 B.C.). On the other hand, *Shen Nong's Herbal Classic*, the earliest materia medica, containing details of usage of various drugs, effectiveness of the herbs from various regions, methods of preparation, preparation prior to usage, and dosages, although attributed to the legendary Shen Nong, was probably written by unknown authors during the western Han dynasty (206 B.C–A.D. 5). This is the first work to summarize all the previous information on Chinese medicinal herbs and is one of the few famous classics on Chinese medicine. It listed 365 drugs, 252 of which were of plant origin, 67 of animal and 46 of mineral origin.

By the 7th century the listing was increased to 844 drugs, as was found in the *Tang Materia Medica*（唐本草）, or the *Newly Compiled Materia Medica of Tang*. This canon consists of 54 volumes and contains descriptions of the plants and their properties, and the flavour of the crude drugs, as well as their therapeutic effects. It was commissioned by the government during the Tang dynasty in A.D. 657, and included plants from the entire country.

The *Tang Materia Medica* was replaced by the *Compendium of Materia Medica*（本草纲目）, published in 1590. Authored by Li Shi Zhen（李时珍）, this major pharmacopoeia of 52 volumes contained 1892 types of drugs, mainly of plant origin, although there were many of animal origin as well as of mineral extraction. This materia medica served China for more than 100 years before extensive revisions and additions were made in the form of Zhao Xue Min's（赵学敏）*Supplement to the Compendium of Materia Medica*（本草纲目拾遗）, published in 1765. More than 900 drugs were recorded in this supplement, bringing the total number of recorded drugs to more than 2500.

With the increase in foreign influence during the Qing dynasty (1644–1911) when Protestant missionaries introduced western medicine, the prestige of Chinese medicine slowly declined. At this juncture, standards of training experienced a decline and the competence of many practitioners was questionable. As a result, Chinese medicine became more and more associated with magic and superstition, and prayers, exorcisms and talismans became important components of the practice. The rural folk still turned to traditional medicine as they could not afford the more modern and expensive western medicine. However, the urban masses and especially the educated viewed it with disfavour. With this decline in prestige, Chinese medical schools gradually closed, one by one.

China moved towards selective modernization around the latter part of the 19th century. During this period more and more physicians were trained in western medicine. Naturally they viewed Chinese medicine with disfavour. This no doubt led to further decline in its prestige. During the Kuomintang era the practitioners of Chinese medicine remained outside the regular medical profession. With the establishment of the People's Republic of China in 1949, Chinese medicine was given official recognition, and it once again came into prominence. Round about 1954, practitioners of Chinese and western medicine were brought together in an effort to get the two groups to work together. The advantage of this move was obvious. With the vast resources of herbal medicine available in the country, it was possible to provide health care to the masses at minimum cost, as opposed to western medicines which required foreign exchange to import. In 1956 the government embarked on a programme to train practitioners of Chinese medicine and during the Great Leap Forward two years later, western-style doctors were also being trained in Chinese medicine.

There were 248 plants and animals listed in *The Atlas of Commonly Used Chinese Traditional Drugs*, prepared in 1970 by the Revolutionary Committee of the Institute of Materia Medica, Chinese Academy of Medical Science, Beijing. The total number of prescriptions, a result of combinations of plants and animals in the atlas, came to 796. These prescriptions are claimed to be commonly used in Chinese medicine today. An evaluation of these prescriptions by the American Herbal Pharmacology delegation to China in 1974 came to the conclusion that 44.7% of them may have a rational basis for their use. This evaluation was done on the basis of the literature reports available then. According to the delegation, this percentage of known or predictably known useful pharmacological effects for Chinese medicines was considerably higher than would result from an analysis of medicinal plants used in the West.

Currently, practitioners of Chinese medicine in China are being given western training and their research institutes are employing modern techniques to validate the efficacy of their medicines. A more applied approach is being attempted, in that, if a drug appears to have beneficial effects, time and money should not be wasted in the isolation of the active properties, and experiments conducted on them.

Chinese medicine is thus actively practised inside China today with full official recognition. It is also practised outside China, in Taiwan, Hong Kong and Singapore, where the population is predominantly ethnic Chinese. The practice is also seen in countries where the population has a significant percentage of ethnic Chinese, like in Malaysia, the Philippines, Thailand or even Indonesia, or anywhere else in the world where there are large pockets of ethnic Chinese, as in Europe and the Americas. Countries such as Japan, Korea and Vietnam also practise this form of health care, although much modified to suit their own national requirements. Most of the raw materials needed by these countries come from China, although Taiwan, and maybe even Hong Kong, may supply some of them. Local materials, where available, may be used as substitutes, or added to the long list of products.

China today is attempting with much success the integration of modern and traditional (Chinese) medical practices. Vietnam similarly has such a programme, run officially by the government. In fact, traditional medicine is taught in a number of national and provincial institutions and also in the faculties of medicine in the universities. South Korea's universities provide formal training in such practices but they do not form part of the official health care service. In Japan practitioners of traditional medicine must first be licensed in modern medicine before they are allowed to practise. Singapore and Malaysia have their own privately run schools to train Chinese medical practitioners, there being no official attempts at integrating at the government hospitals.

In most of these cultures, Chinese medicine, or a variation of it, is very much accepted by a large percentage of the population. Many of these people still believe they can be properly cured by the traditional practitioners. This does not mean that they shun modern medicine. Many, in fact, view the two practices as complementary, consulting one for certain ailments and the other for others, or even alternating from one to the other, if it is thought that one system is not providing the necessary relief.

With such wide following, this form of alternate medicine should not be totally dismissed. Through the centuries many of these crude drugs of herbal origin, be they used in Chinese, Indian, American or European traditional medicines, have been shown to be effective, with real therapeutic values. Although critics may say that this has been the result of years of trial and error, the fact remains that many of the drugs have been effective in curing various ailments, although many have since proved to be totally useless. Those that have been proved to be of value include ephedrin, obtained from *ma huang*, or *Ephedra*, now used to treat asthma, just as it was centuries ago.

Another example is digitalis, one of the most important heart medications, extracted from *mao di huang* or foxglove (*Digitalis purpurea*), another traditional Chinese medicine. This plant has, together with some 20 other plants, also been used for centuries in England to treat dropsy, a condition resulting from the inefficient working of the heart, causing a general swelling of the body. However, it was only in 1785 that the active ingredient of this herbal treatment was narrowed down to the leaves of the foxglove. Two drugs isolated from this plant, digoxin and digitoxin, are now official drugs in the British as well as other pharmacopoeias. Foxglove leaves are used worldwide today by many doctors as a remedy for congestive heart failure, in preference to the pure drugs, which are deemed more dangerous.

The roots of *Rauvolfia serpentina* have been used for centuries in traditional Indian medicine to treat the mentally ill. Similarly, African traditional medicine uses the African species, *R. vomitoria*, for the same purpose. Subsequent research unearthed the presence of many alkaloids, such as reserpine, rescinamine and deserpidine, in these plants. Reserpine, together with some others, has tranquilizing and antihypertensive properties, and is used in modern medicine today.

Harmony

The Chinese believe that two basic and opposing principles, *yin* and *yang*, govern the universe and all phenomena result from their continuous interplay. *Yin* (阴) is represented by feminity, darkness, cold and water, *yang* (阳) by masculinity, sun, heat and fire. Individually, we are dominated by one of the two elements and should eat and drink chiefly things which help maintain the balance. When the *yin/yang* equilibrium is disturbed, illness results; herbs are prescribed to redress this imbalance.

Chinese Herbs and their preparation

Chinese herbs are not merely dried plant parts or animals. In many cases they are actually crude drugs, while some have been specially processed to enhance the quality of the basic material. Most of the herbs used are never used alone. Rather, they are used together with others, to make up a prescription. In Chinese medicine, there are more than 100 different prescriptions in general use today. The actual combination in quantities and in the number of ingredients in each prescription may vary from one practitioner to another, but, generally, the main ingredients remain the same. Also, the quantity of each ingredient may vary, depending on the practitioner's assessment of the patient's health, his sex as well as his weight.

The practitioner usually diagnoses the ailment before offering a prescription. The patient is questioned regarding the aches and pains he experiences, his general appetite, how he feels, and so on. The practitioner also uses his power of observation to note the patient's skin colour, texture, redness of nose, etc. Smells, especially body odour, also provide clues to the condition of the various organs such as stomach, lungs, liver, kidney, bladder and colon. Touching of the patient is also involved, in particular, to read his pulse, and to palpate his abdomen as well as the diagnostic acupuncture points.

A prescription usually involves a main ingredient and many supporting ingredients, the latter playing varying roles from preserving and flavouring to colouring. Herbs are usually prescribed as a decoction. This needs preparation as the herbal mixture needs to be boiled over a low fire in an enamel or earthernware container in twice the required amount of water. Once the volume of the mixture has been reduced by half, the decoction is poured off and drunk when sufficiently cooled. The remaining herbal mixture in the container can be reused once. Boiling allows the drugs to be dissolved into the water and sometimes for any toxic substances, which can cause side effects, to be deactivated. It also has the advantage of sterilizing the mixture.

Herbs can also be prescribed as powder or pill. In the case of the former, the mixture is ground and dissolved in hot or warm water. Pills are the most convenient to take as they come in ready-to-swallow forms. Usually, a pill is bound with honey or jujube meat to give it an agreeable flavour. Ointment can also be made by boiling the drugs until the liquid thickens, when sugar is added to get a thick paste. This form is mainly used for external applications.

In a medically advanced world, one may rightly ask what the advantages are of taking Chinese medicine in comparison with modern scientific medicine. Many practitioners of Chinese medicine believe that both have a role to play in modern society. Drugs are fast-acting, thus very useful in severe conditions of illness. On the other hand herbs are slow-acting and never extremely potent. They are thus suitable for many chronic illnesses where a slow approach to treatment is desirable. The crude drugs, the processed herbs, release their active ingredients slowly in the system. Also, the presence of other substances may slow the absorption or may enhance the absorption of the active ingredients. It has also been shown that the active ingredients in a herb may have a different effect from the pure form. Ephedrine increases the blood pressure and heart beat when given for asthma. However, when the plant ephedra is used, no side effects are seen. Another example is seen in the use of foxglove: a lower dosage is needed to treat heart condition when using the extract, digitalis. Using the plant produces nausea as a result of side effects while the pure chemical interferes with the normal rhythm of the heart.

How to Use this Book
The plants treated in this book are arranged in alphabetical order according to their generic names which are given at the top of each section. Below the generic name is the botanical family the plant belongs to, after which comes the scientific name. The scientific name is made up of two parts: the generic name followed by the specific name. By convention the scientific name is written in italics or underlined. Very often, the generic name is of Latin or Greek origin, but Latinized, as Latin is accepted as the universal botanical language in the naming of plants. As far as possible, the origin of the generic name is given in the text. The specific name is usually adjectival but again Latinized. It can describe the habit of the plant, the size or shape of an organ, the origin of the plant, the country where it was first described or, sometimes, be named after a particular person.

The Chinese name is also given, together with the common name/s of the herb. As with common names, there are often more than one per plant and different countries may use different common names. Confusion can arise as a result of using common names, thus more than one are given in the text. An index of common names is given at the end of the book for readers to trace a particular plant based on the common name. However, there is no guarantee that all common names are recorded here – only the more common ones.

Each entry includes information of the plant itself – the origin of the scientific and common names where available, a brief description of the plant, interesting anecdotes, as well as its usage other than its usage in Chinese medicine, which is given at the end of the section, according to the different parts of the plant.

However, where more than one species of a genus is treated within each section, only the generic name is given, below the family, after which come the common names for the genus where available. The main entry gives information about the genus. The different species of the genus follow the main entry, with the scientific names, Chinese and common names where available, a short description where necessary, and medicinal usage.

For each plant there are numerous uses, varying from practitioner to practitioner, and from country to country. Only a few are listed for each plant as it would not be possible to list them all.

ABRUS
Family: Leguminosae

Abrus precatorius 相思子
rosary pea
love pea
Indian licorice
wild licorice vine
weather plant
weather vine
prayer-beads
coral-bead plant
red-bead vine
crab's-eye
precatory bean

The plant is a delicate climber native to the tropics but now widely naturalized. The seeds are tiny, glossy and hard, and scarlet in colour, with a jet black base. They are harmless when whole and intact but highly poisonous when cracked. A single cracked seed, when swallowed, can cause death in a man. Thus they can be very dangerous when made into trinkets such as necklaces, rosaries and bangles, especially when the individual seeds get into the hands of children. The generic name, *Abrus*, is Greek for delicate, in reference to the small leaflets, while the common names mainly refer to the attractive seeds.

Parts used:
seeds: treat fever, malaria, headache, dropsy; expel intestinal worms

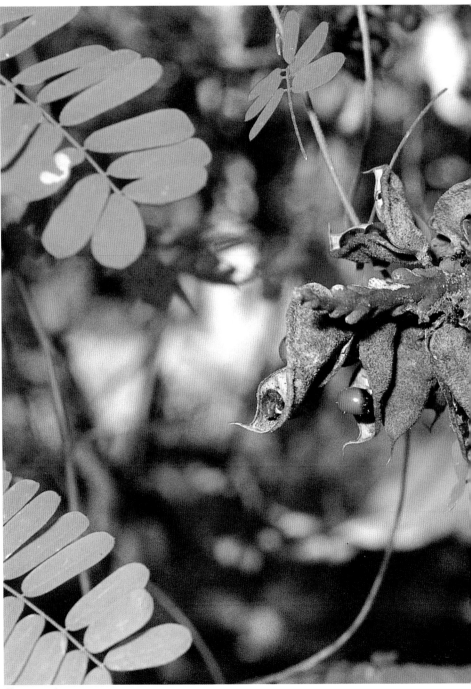

Abrus precatorius

14

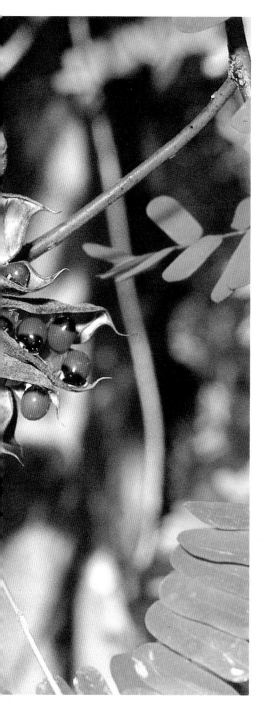

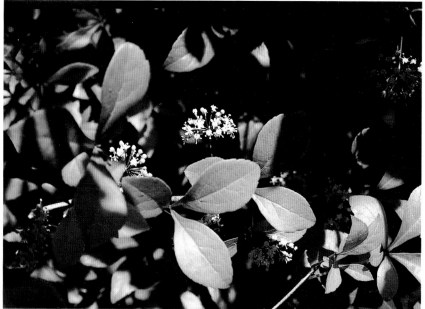

Acanthopanax gracilistylus

ACANTHOPANAX
Family: Araliaceae
Acanthopanax
spiny panax

Acanthopanax is derived from the Greek words *akantha*, "thorn", *pan*, "all", and *akes*, "remedy". The plant is thus a thorny panax, or panacea. These small trees, many of which are deciduous, are native to East Asia, the Malay Peninsula and the Philippine Islands.

Acanthopanax gracilistylus 五加
Parts used:
bark of the roots: tonic for general weakness; treats rheumatism, impotence, lumbago, syphilis

Acanthopanax davidii
Parts used:
whole plant: treats mechanical injury

Acanthopanax trifoliatus 白苈
Parts used:
stem: wash for leprosy
leaves: tonic; treat tuberculosis, partial paralysis, bleeding in the lungs

15

ACONITUM
Family: Ranunculaceae
Aconitum
monkshood

These are north temperate herbs with purplish, reddish-purple or white flowers and thickened roots. They are also called aconite or, scientifically, *Aconitum*; the root word is derived from the Greek *akon*, meaning "dart". The name monkshood comes from the shape of the flower, which resembles the cowl of the Benedictine monks. Many of these plants are highly poisonous, due to the presence, in the roots and leaves, of an alkaloid aconitine, and, perhaps, other alkaloids as well. According to Greek mythology, the poison of the monkshood was the foam that dripped from the mouth of the three-headed dog, Cerebus, when Hercules, performing his twelfth labour, dragged it from Hades. Wherever the spittle of the dog spilled, these plants sprouted.

The juice of certain monkshood was used in ancient times to poison wells and springs, usually by a retreating population, in the face of an invading enemy. The poison was also favoured for use among the common people in ancient Europe, while those of the higher class had a preference for hemlock; a decoction of the

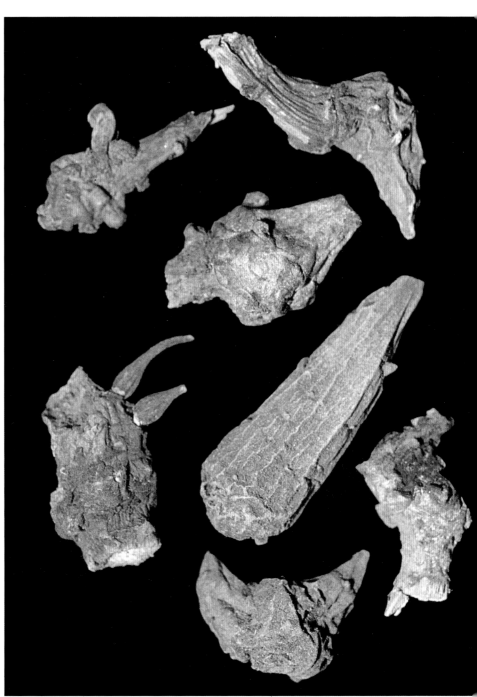

Aconitum transectum

roots was given to criminals to end their life. On the Greek island of Ceos, the infirm old were forced to take aconite.

Another use of monkshood was in the concoction, together with deadly nightshade, of the so-called "flying ointment", believed to be used by witches to enable them to fly. It is now believed that a combination of these two plant drugs could impart the sensation of flight to anyone under their influence.

The drug aconite, available in Chinese pharmacies, represents the underground stems of several species of the plant. The fresh parts are extremely poisonous but not the dried ones, for drying changes much of the toxic alkaloid to a less toxic compound. This drug has been in use in China, probably for more than 2000 years.

Aconitum carmichaelii 乌头
Aconitum chinensis 中国乌头
Aconitum transectum 直缘乌头
Parts used:
underground stem: stimulant; heart tonic; pain killer; narcotic; mild laxative; local anaesthetic; treats colds, chills, vomiting, rheumatoid arthritis, chest pain, stomachache, loss of appetite, inflammation of the kidney

Aconitum vulparia
Parts used:
underground stem: narcotic

AGASTACHE
Family: Labiatae
Agastache rugosa
wrinkled giant hyssop 藿香

The generic name *Agastache* is Greek for "many-spiked", referring to the flowering spikes of this tall herb. The plant is native to China, Japan, northern Vietnam and Laos, and is cultivated in China. The sweetish and highly aromatic leaves are medicinal and may be used together with the stems and roots. Experiments have shown the leaves to have antitumour properties when tested on animals. Outside China the plant has been used to treat cancer.

Parts used:
whole plant: treats fever, headache, vomiting, diarrhoea, nausea, excessive gas in the system, colds, indigestion, cholera

AGRIMONIA
Family: Rosaceae
Agrimonia
agrimony

The plant is a light, aromatic, hairy herb, less than 2 m tall, and native to Europe and western Asia. It has lobed leaves, with the basal ones arranged in a rosette, while those along the stem are

alternately placed. Flowers are golden-yellow, small, and in loose, long bunches, the individual flowers opening from the base of the bunch upwards. The generic name, *Agrimonia*, comes from the Greek *agremone*, formerly misinterpreted as meaning "a white speck in the eye", for which the plant was said to be a cure. There are others who believe that the name in Latin means "defender of the field", as the plant grows around the edge of fields. It is a source of a golden-yellow dye.

Besides being used by the Chinese, this plant is also widely used in European and American herbal treatments. The Zulus drink a decoction of the leaves to expel tapeworms.

Agrimonia eupatoria 欧产仙鹤草
Parts used:
stems, leaves: treat vomiting of blood, dysentery, blood in the urine and in the stools, bleeding of the uterus, pain in the stomach, exhaustion from overwork
roots: heart tonic; treat tuberculosis

Agrimonia pilosa 疏毛龙芽草
Parts used:
whole plant: treats vomiting of blood, dysentery, blood in the urine and in stools, bleeding of the uterus, pain in the stomach, exhaustion from overwork

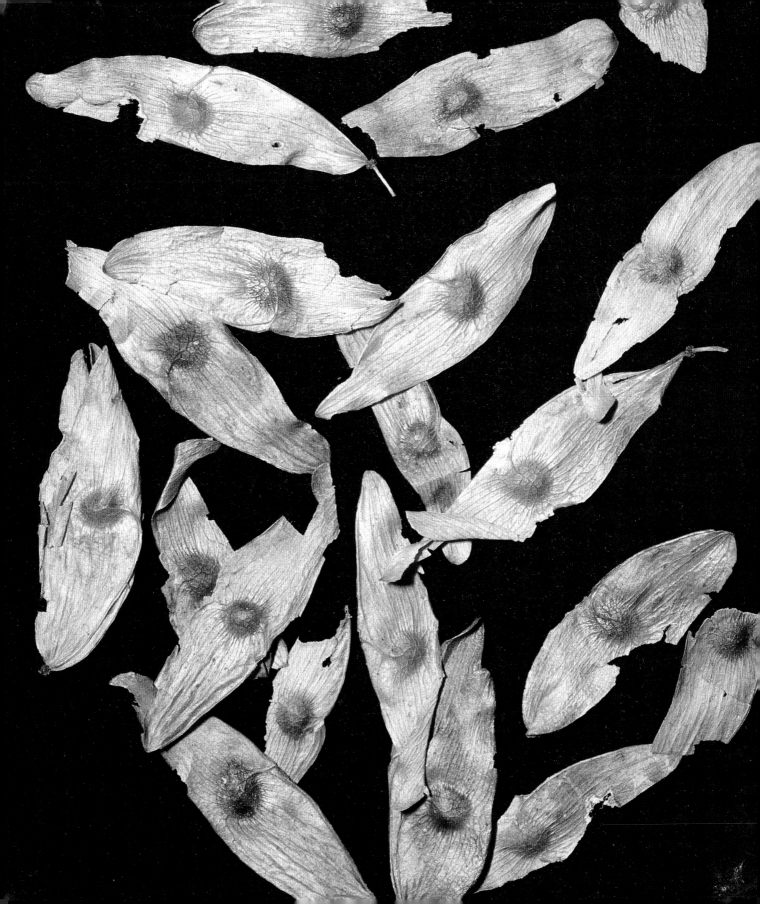

AILANTHUS
Family: Simaroubaceae
Ailanthus altissima 臭椿
tree-of-heaven
varnish tree
copal tree

This is a fast growing tree, native to China. The female tree is commonly planted as an ornament but not the male tree because the small, greenish male flowers give off a sweetish to foetid smell. The leaves give off a foul smell when crushed. Fruits are two-winged, twisted, and turn reddish-orange when ripe. The leaves were once used as a yellow dye for wool, as well as to make paper.

Parts used:
root bark, fruits: treat dysentery, vaginal discharge, piles, bloody stools, premature ejaculation; expel tapeworms; increase menstrual flow

AKEBIA
Family: Lardizabalaceae
Akebia quinata 木通
five-leaf akebia
chocolate vine

This is an attractive woody climber, native to Japan, China and Korea. The plant bears purplish young branches and bunches of fragrant, purplish flowers. The stem is medicinal. It is available from Chinese pharmacies as thin slices, each slice having a prominent centre full of holes.

Parts used:
stem: purgative; treats inflammation of the skin, fever; induces secretion of milk in women after birth; increases menstrual flow; induces sweating
fruit stalk: purgative
roots: treat fever

ALBIZIA
Family: Leguminosae
Albizia julibrissin 合欢
mimosa tree
silk tree

The tall and wide-spreading tree is a popular ornamental tree, native to regions extending from Iran to Japan, and now naturalized in many countries.

Parts used:
bark: tranquilizer; relieves pain; improves blood circulation; treats insomnia, lung cancer, fractures, bleedings
flowers: tonic

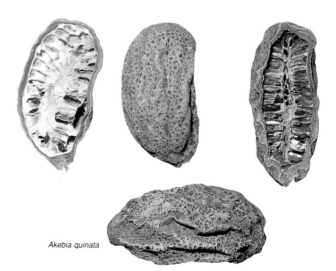

Akebia quinata

ALEURITES
Family: Euphorbiaceae
Aleurites fordii 油桐
tung oil tree
China wood-oil tree

The name *Aleurites* is Greek for farinose, or floury. This is a central Asian tree, now cultivated in a number of countries as a source of tung-oil, used in paints and quick-drying varnishes. Lamp black for the making of Indian ink comes from tung-oil. The fruit kernel is poisonous and cases of poisoning from eating them have been reported. Both the seed oil and the plant have insecticidal properties.

Parts used:
oil: treats boils, ulcers, swellings, burns, scalds
immature fruits: treat anaemia resulting in an absence of menstruation

ALISMA
Family:Alismataceae
Alisma plantago-aquatica 泽泻
water plantain
mad-dog weed

This is a marshy herb, native to North America and temperate East Asia. Research on this plant has shown that it has anticancer property and is also capable of inducing an abnormally low sugar content in the blood of animals.

Parts used:
underground stem: treats high blood pressure, diabetes, kidney inflammation, painful urination, venereal diseases, vertigo, lumbago, premature ejaculation; induces secretion of milk in women who have just given birth; increases flow of urine

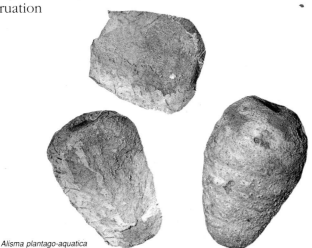

Alisma plantago-aquatica

ALLIUM
Family: Amaryllidaceae
Allium sativum 大蒜
garlic

The generic name, *Allium*, is the Latin name for the plant, which is of European origin. It has an ovoid to roundish bulb which is usually divided into several cloves, each enclosed within a membraneous coat. The flowering stalk bears leaves towards the lower end and a small bunch of flowers at the top. The pinkish flowers are on long stalks. The plant is widely cultivated as a condiment for the flavouring of foods particularly in countries bordering the Mediterranean. In the days of ancient Greece and Rome, garlic was popularly consumed by the working class, but not the upper class as it was then considered vulgar to exhale the characteristic odour. In medieval Europe it was widely used to disguise the smell and flavour of salted meat and fish. The green tops as well as the bulbs are consumed in tropical countries.

The medicinal value of garlic has been recognized since early times. The Egyptians have been using garlic as a cure for headache, worms, tumours and even heart problems for more than 3000 years. Dioscorides, the chief physician to the Roman army in the first century

A.D., prescribed garlic to expel intestinal worms. Athletes ate garlic during the first Olympic games in Greece to give them added energy. Garlic is also recognized as a powerful antidote against all kinds of poisons. There are reports that garlic prevents the occurrence of cancer; how else can one explain the low incidence of the disease among the garlic-eating French?

In Chinese medicine the use of garlic has been traced to the reign of Emperor Huang Di, when some of his followers were cured of plant poisoning by the use of wild garlic. The bulbs have the reputation as an all-purpose healing agent.

Parts used:
bulbs: treat asthma, bronchitis, cold, diarrhoea, tuberculosis, abscesses; remove excessive gas in the system; expel phlegm from the respiratory passages; expel intestinal worms

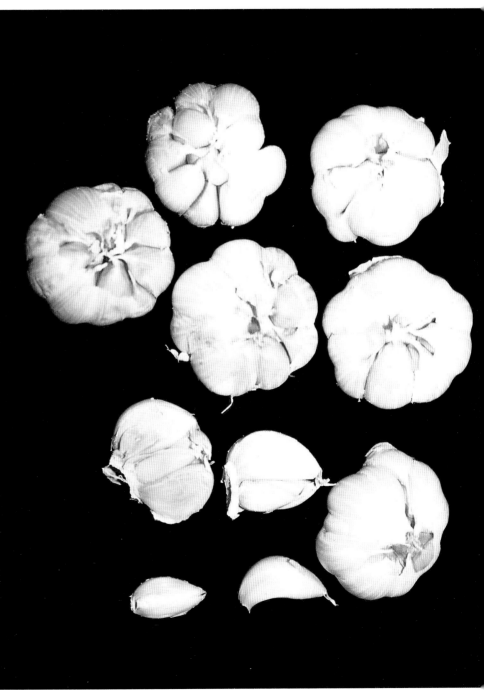

Allium sativum

21

ALOE
Family:Liliaceae
Aloe barbadensis (= A. vera)
库拉索芦荟
medicinal aloe
Barbados aloe

The aloe is a plant of the arid regions of the Old World. It is a stemless, succulent herb, with thick, hard, sharp-pointed leaves in a close rosette. The flowers arise from a long stalk growing from the centre of the rosette of leaves, usually very much higher than the plant itself. It is supposed to originate from the Mediterranean regions but is now widely cultivated as an ornament or as a source of the drug aloe. The plant is currently extensively used in many cosmetic and medicinal preparations for the treatment of pimples, acne, mouth ulcers and insect bites; to arrest bleeding and itching of piles; and as a temporary relief from arthritic pains.

Parts used:
juice from leaves: mild laxative; wash for piles; treats abscesses, scabies; increases menstrual flow

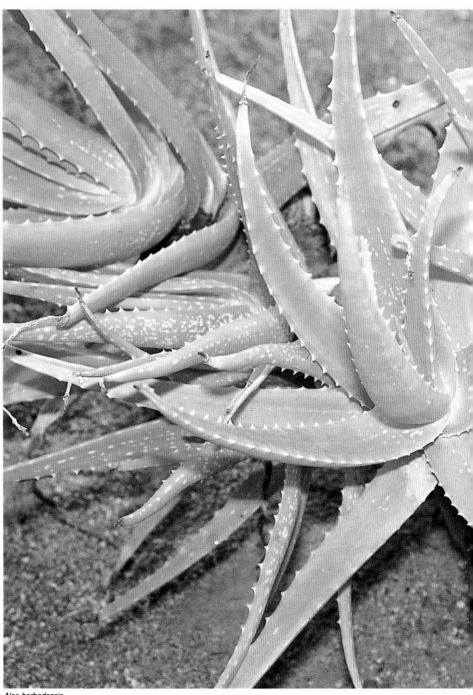

Aloe barbadensis

22

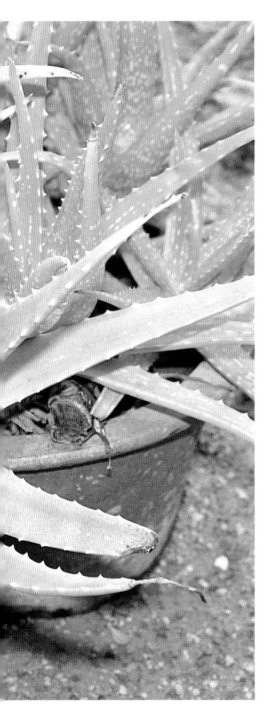

AMOMUM
Family: Zingiberaceae
Amomum compactum
round cardamom

Round cardamom is a large herb, native to Java. The seeds are spicy and aromatic, and are sometimes used as a substitute for the true cardamom. Besides being used by the Chinese, it is also used by the Malays and the Indonesians.

Parts used:
fruits: stimulate gastric activities; prevent vomiting; expel gas from system

AMORPHOPHALLUS
Family: Araceae
Amorphophallus rivieri 魔芋
devil's tongue
snake palm

The plant is a gigantic herb of the Old World tropics. The underground stem produces a single huge leaf made up of a trunk-like stalk at the end of which is the much-divided leaf blade. The production of the leaf is followed by an immense, hooded flowering stalk bearing numerous unisexual flowers. This structure emits a strong, disagreeable odour. The underground stems are sliced, washed to remove the toxic substances, dried and powdered to be made into a food resembling beancurd. The Japanese produces a vermicelli from it.

Parts used:
stem: treats poisonous snake bites
flowering stalk: reduces fever

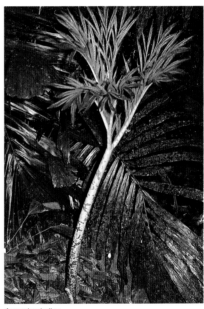

Amorphophallus

23

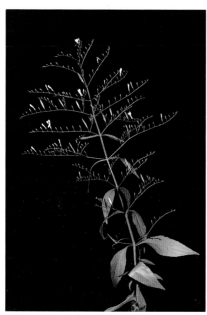
Andrographis paniculata

AMPELOPSIS
Family: Vitaceae
Ampelopsis japonica 白蔹
ampelopsis

This is native to China and Japan. As the name *Ampelopsis*, which is Greek for "vine-like", implies, the plant is a woody vine. It is a deciduous plant which climbs with the help of tendrils.

Parts used:
roots: anticonvulsant; purgative; cooling agent; expel phlegm; treat inflammation of the skin, burns, boils, ulcers, acne, swellings, vaginal and uterine discharges

ANDROGRAPHIS
Family: Acanthaceae
Andrographis paniculata 穿心莲
creat

This Asian herb grows as a weed from India, southwards through Thailand and Peninsular Malaysia, to Indonesia.

Parts used:
whole plant: treats influenza, bronchitis, pneumonia, whooping cough, gall bladder infection, high blood pressure, burns, bites

ANEMARRHENA
Family: Liliaceae
Anemarrhena asphodeloides 知母
anemarrhena

This plant, a herb with grass-like leaves, is native to north China. The underground stem is used in small doses to treat various ailments. However, in large doses it is said to be toxic, inhibiting the action of the heart. Extracts of the plant have yielded steroidal saponins, which contain an anti-inflammatory property, thus its use in the treatment of lumbago.

Parts used:
underground stem: calms thirst in fever; treats congestive fever, excessive sweating, dry throat, hacking cough, dizziness, lumbago, pneumonia, morning sickness, measles, premature ejaculation

ANEMONE
Family: Ranunculaceae
Anemone
anemone

Anemones are herbs, native to temperate areas. All are poisonous, as is evidenced in the use of the plant extracts to poison arrow tips in Kamchatka, USSR. The sap can cause irritation of the skin, resulting in painful blisters. Taken internally, the plant may result in acute inflammation of the digestive tracts and kidneys. In severe cases cramps, unconsciousness and even death through respiratory failure may result. The poison is glycoside ranunculin.

Anemone hupehensis var. *japonica* 变种秋牡丹
Japanese anemone
Parts used:
whole plant: treats ringworm, tuberculosis of the lymphatic glands

Anemone cernua
Parts used:
roots: treat bone fracture, stomachache, toothache, aching bones, sore throat

Anemone chinensis 白头翁
Parts used:
roots: treat diarrhoea

Anemone raddena 红背银莲花
Parts used:
roots: treat swelling, itch, skin
rash

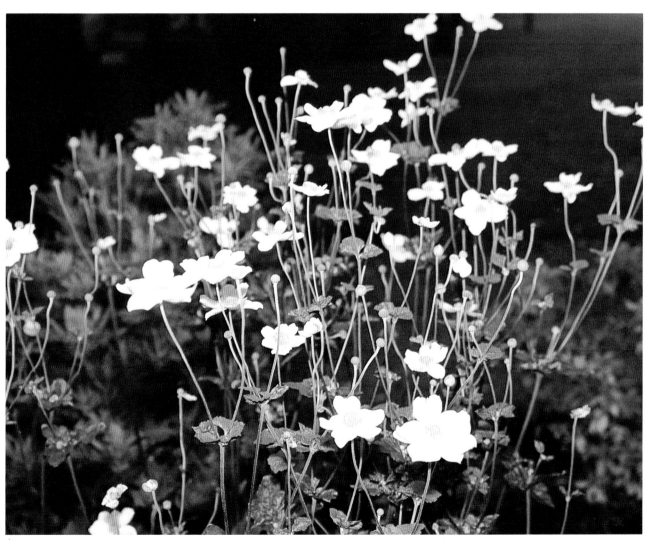

Anemone

Anemone

25

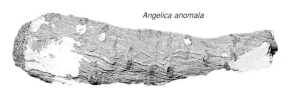
Angelica anomala

ANGELICA
Family: Umbelliferae
Angelica
angelica
holy ghost plant
holy plant
root of the holy ghost

Angelica was believed to be of heavenly origin, its healing properties made known to a monk in a dream, thus its generic name. According to one legend, the plant was revealed in a dream by an angel to cure the plague. The virtues of *Angelica archangelica*, commonly known as archangel, were extolled by old writers in Europe who testified to its usefulness in curing every conceivable disease. Its specific name (not to mention the generic name) bears testimony to the faith people placed in the plant. It is said to bloom on the Feast of the Apparition of St Michael, the Archangel, thus it is believed to ward off witchcraft and evil spirits.

Angelica is largely used as a flavouring for confectionery and liqueurs. It is also used for medicine and in perfumery. Many western herbalists since time immemorial have a high regard for angelica, using it as a protection against contagious diseases as well as a cure for almost every disease.

Angelica sinensis 当归
Parts used:
roots: tonic; sedative; purgative; stimulate blood circulation; increase the flow of urine; treat difficult, painful or absence of menstruation, constipation

Angelica anomala 川白芷
Angelica dahurica 兴安白芷
Parts used:
roots: pain killer for use in common cold, headache and fever; treat boils and abscesses, itching, diptheria, blood in the urine, snake bites, vaginal discharge

Angelica pubescens 重齿毛当归
Parts used:
roots: treat nose bleed, blood in urine, rheumatic arthritis, lumbago, common cold, headache; increase menstrual flow

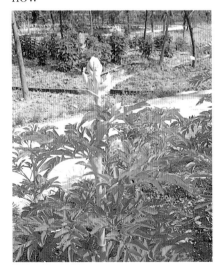
Angelica

AQUILARIA
Family: Thymelaeaceae
Aquilaria
eagle-wood tree

Aquilaria, from the Latin *aquila*, "eagle", is a genus of tropical trees valued for the fragrant, resin-infiltrated wood known commercially as eagle-wood or aloes wood. To the Malays it is known as *gaharu*, which is a corruption of the Sanskritic *agaru*. This wood is sought after in the East, where it is used as incense and in native medicines. The fragrant wood only develops when the trees are dying, supposedly as a result of a fungal infection. With infection, dark, hard and fragrant lumps develop, embedded within the normal wood. These pieces are harvested by chopping down the tree and splitting the trunk lengthwise. So valuable is this eagle-wood or aloes wood that large-scale destruction of perfectly healthy trees in the forests have made the eagle-wood trees an endangered species.

The resinous wood was formerly imported into China for medicinal purposes. The grated wood is included in preparations used to treat rheumatism, smallpox and illness during and after childbirth.

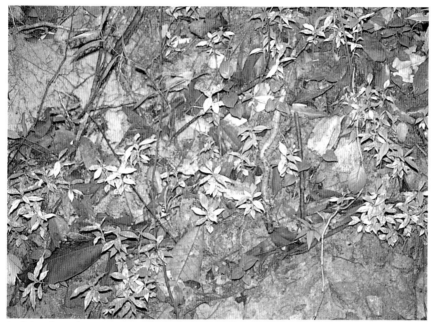

Aquilaria malaccensis

Aquilaria malaccensis 沉香
Malayan eagle-wood tree
kayu gaharu
The grated wood was formerly imported into China.

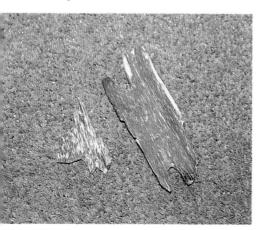

Aquilaria malaccensis

Parts used:
wood: stimulant; aphrodisiac; tonic; diuretic; expels gas from system

Aquilaria sinensis 白木香
This is a tree of southeastern China, now replacing the Malayan eagle-wood tree for medicinal purposes. The Chinese collectors inflict wounds on the tree to induce the secretion of resins which are regularly collected. The wounds subsequently heal and the wood around the old wounds is cut off for use. This in turn causes the formation of new wounds and more resin is secreted, and so the process is repeated. Alternatively, a gap is made on the trunk by chiselling away at the wood and the space thus formed filled with clay; the resin that flows out from the wound accumulates in the clay. Old and dying trees are cut down and the trunks sliced for the heartwood which is also used medicinally.

Parts used:
resinous wood, resin: tonic for the kidneys; expel gas; treat male disorders, shortness of breath, nausea, general pains, weak knees, chills, chest and abdominal pains, asthma

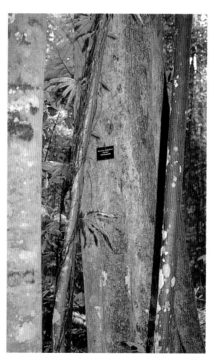

Aquilaria malaccensis

ARCTIUM
Family: Compositae
Arctium lappa 牛蒡
great burdock
edible burdock
cuckold

The name *Arctium* is derived from the Greek *arctos*, meaning "bear", alluding to the rough, furry texture of the bracts around the flowers. The specific name, *lappa*, comes from the Celtic *llap*, "hand", in reference to the hooked bracts which attach themselves to passing animals which assist in their dispersal. This is a weed with large leaves, found on wasteland and by waysides in Asia and Europe. Flowers are purple and in roundish heads around the ends of branches. Bracts surrounding the flowers end in sharp hooks. These hooks attach themselves to passing animals causing the snapping of the stem. This in turn helps to eject the ripe fruits from the fruiting head onto animals which thus assist in their dispersal.

The plant has a long history of being used as an antibacterial folk remedy outside China. The American Indians and the Europeans also use it for various ailments. The plant was an important ingredient in a cure for stones in the gall bladder and kidney during the Middle Ages. The roots yield an oil that was once used to treat baldness and skin disorders.

Parts used:
leaves: treat dizziness, rheumatism
fruits, seeds: treat common cold, pneumonia, sore throat, smallpox, scarlet fever, constipation, pimples, skin infection called St Anthony's fire, mumps, early symptoms of measles
roots: mild laxative; induce sweating; induce flow of urine

ARECA
Family: Palmae
Areca catechu 槟榔
areca nut
betel nut
betel palm
pinang
catechu

The handsome palm has a solitary, slender stem, growing sometimes to a height of more than 25 m. Male and female

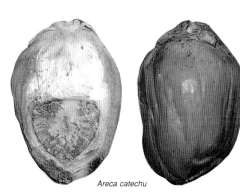

Areca catechu

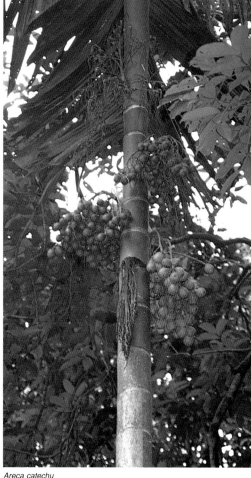

Areca catechu

flowers are found on the same tree; the former are few and on the lower part of the flowering stalk. Fruits are oval, about 5 cm long, and orange to red in colour, with a soft and fibrous outer covering enclosing a hard seed. The exact origin of this palm is not known but it is generally believed that it came from the Malay Peninsula. The palm is widely planted throughout the Old World tropics, where the kernel is an important masticatory. The kernel is chewed as a narcotic,

28

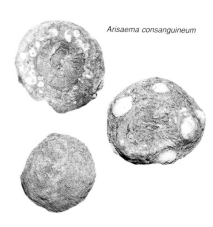

Arisaema consanguineum

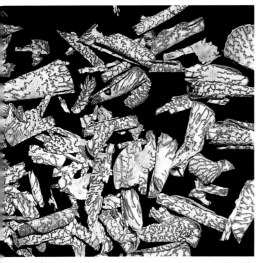

reca catechu

fresh or cured with slacked lime, betel leaves and various other spices as flavourings. The quid is retained in the mouth and chewed slowly. This results in continuous salivation; the saliva, stained bright red, is spat out. The quid is similarly spat out eventually.

Parts used:
ripe seed: treats diarrhoea, indigestion, lumbago, urinary problems; expels tapeworms and roundworms; increases menstrual flow

ARISAEMA
Family: Araceae
Arisaema
arisaema

The name *Arisaema* is derived from the Greek words, *aris* and *haema*, meaning "arum" and "blood", referring to the red-blotched leaves of some species. A number of species of these stemless, tuberous herbs are used in Chinese medicine. Certain species have been shown to have anti-cancer property when tested on animals. Use of other species by non-Chinese traditional medicines include treatments for fever, inflammation, cancer, fungal infection, infertility, as a pain killer, and to increase the flow of urine.

Arisaema amurense 东北天南星
Arisaema consanguineum 天南星
Arisaema heterophyllum 异叶天南星
Arisaema japonicum 鬼蒟蒻
Parts used:
underground stem: treats cough, dizziness, epilepsy, convulsions in children, blood poisoning, tetanus, inflammation of the liver and pancreas, snake bites

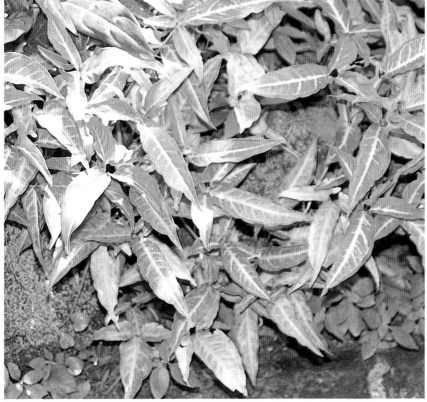

Arisaema

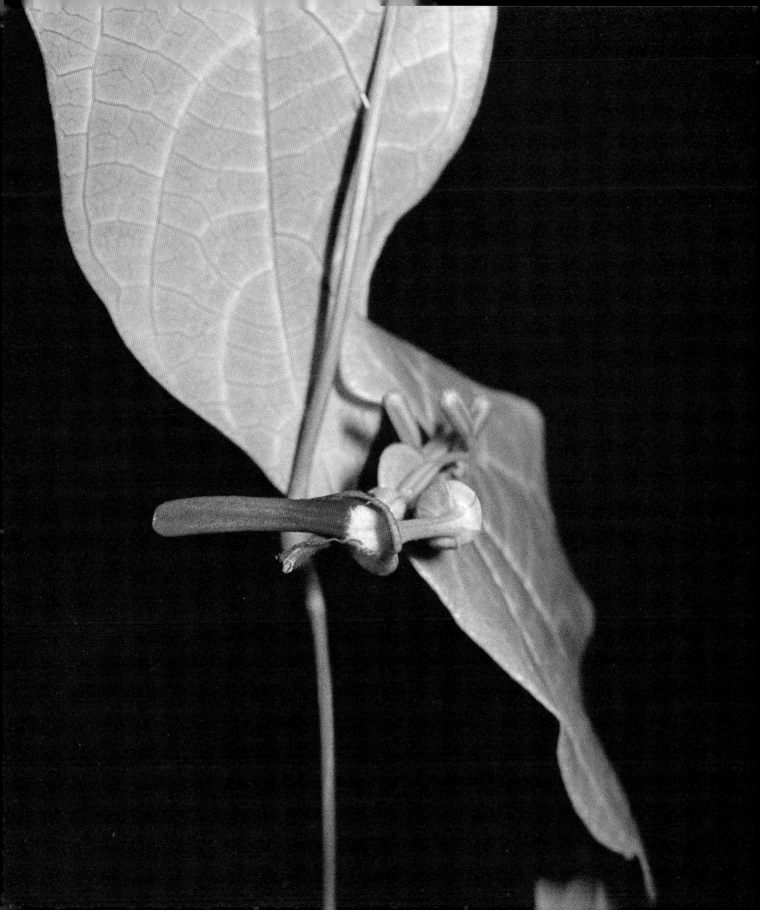

ARISTOLOCHIA
Family: Aristolochiaceae
Aristolochia
birthworts
Dutchman's pipe

Birthworts are native to northern China and Japan. They are so called because of their use by herbalists to remove obstructions after birth as well as to treat difficult births. Their curved flowers, looking very much like a womb, no doubt contribute to such usage. Its other name, Dutchman's pipe, needs no explanation. The generic name, *Aristolochia*, comes from the Greek words *aristos* and *locheia*, meaning "noblest" and "childbirth", referring to its supposed medicinal properties. The fruit resembles the human lung and has thus been used in pulmonary disorders such as asthma, bronchitis and coughs. The plant has also been used in Indian, American and European folk medicines.

Aristolochic acid, present in most species, is poisonous, causing serious disorders of the digestive tract, inflammation of the kidneys, and miscarriage. A poisonous alkaloid has also been isolated from the fruits which, at high dosage, causes cardiac and respiratory arrests in experimental animals. A species present in South America is used as an arrow poison, while

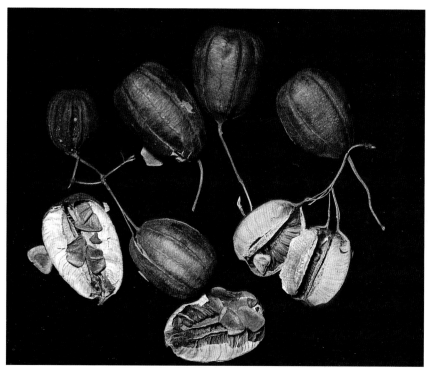

Aristolochia debilis

another in East Africa is poisonous to cattle. At least 20 species of *Aristolochia* have been used for cancer remedies in folk medicine. However, while aristolochic acid has been shown to be an active antitumour agent in animals, it is too toxic for clinical use.

Aristolochia debilis 马兜铃
Aristolochia contorta 北马兜铃
Parts used:
leaves, roots: treat indigestion with pain in the stomach, high blood pressure, diarrhoea, dysentery, insect bite poisoning; antidote for snake poisoning

stem: stimulates circulation of the blood; relieves pain; induces flow of urine
fruit: antidote for snake poisoning

Aristolochia manshuriensis
木通马兜铃
Parts used:
stem: treats fever, diabetes; increases flow of urine; induces menstruation; stimulates milk flow in women after labour

Aristolochia westlandii 白金果榄
Parts used:
roots: treat rashes, itch, swollen feet, beri-beri, aches, numbness

31

ARTEMISIA
Family: Compositae
Artemisia
mugwort
sagebrush
wormwood
wormseed

Mugworts are aromatic perennial herbs, usually grown as ornaments and for their medicinal and aromatic qualities. Flowers are small and grouped in compact heads which are reddish brown in colour. The entire plant has a characteristic odour. It is also known as wormseed as the seeds are used to expel intestinal worms. But the genus is named after the Greek goddess Artemisia.

Artemisia vulgaris 野艾
The leaves are used as a condiment and as a bitter in certain alcoholic beverages. They are medicinal as well, containing the chemical artemisin, which is bitter to taste.

Parts used:
leaves: relieve headache; treat swellings and sprains, asthma, menstrual disorders; stimulate gastric activities; stop bleeding

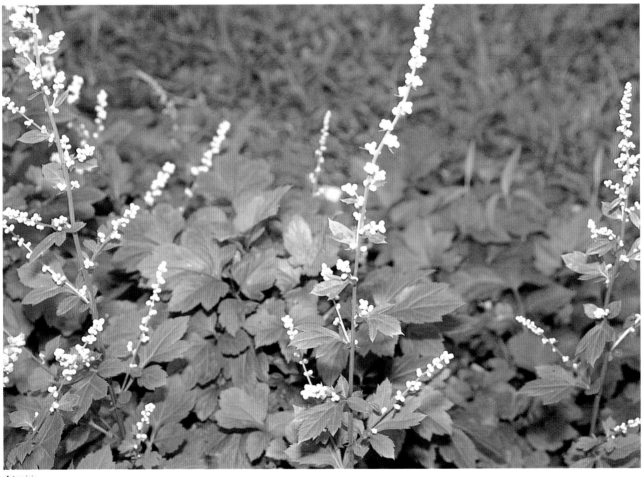

Artemisia

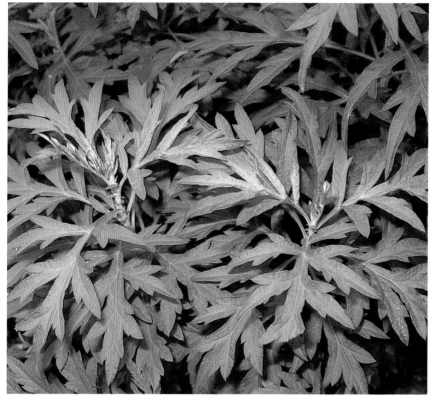
Artemisia vulgaris

Artemisia annua 黄花蒿
sweet wormwood
Parts used:
seeds: treat sweating at night, indigestion, eye diseases
leaf stalks: treat chronic dysentery, eye diseases

Artemisia capillaris 茵陈蒿
This species is a purplish-looking herb, native to northern China, Japan and Taiwan. The plant contains an essential oil which has been shown to have antifungal and antibacterial properties.

Parts used:
young plants: cool the body system; treat infectious hepatitis, jaundice, constipation, fever; increase flow of urine

Artemisia apiacea 青蒿
Parts used:
whole plant: reduces fever; stops bleeding; treats dysentery, malaria, dizziness, night sweating, nose bleeding
flowers: treat rheumatism, lumbago, headache

Artemisia argyi 艾
Parts used:
leaves: treat excessive bleeding during menstruation, bleeding during pregnancy or after labour, bleeding of the nose, vomiting of blood, blood in stools, diarrhoea
leaf stalks: treat chronic dysentery, eye disease
seeds: treat sweating at night, excessive gas in the system, tuberculosis, indigestion

ASARUM
Family: Aristolochiaceae
Asarum sieboldii 华细辛
wild ginger

The generic name *Asarum* comes from the Greek word *asaron*, which is the name of the asarabacca, a low, stemless shrub. This is a north temperate plant, native to northern China and Japan. It has an underground stem which bears hairy, heart-shaped leaves on a long stalk. Flowers are reddish, solitary and occur near the surface of the ground.

Parts used:
whole plant: treats common cold, headache, toothache, vomiting, chronic bronchitis, coughs, ulcers on the tongue and in the mouth
roots: pain killer; sedative; remove excessive gas in the system; treat pulmonary related disorders

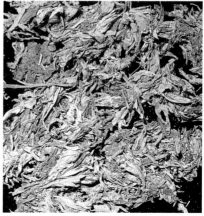
Artemisia

ASPARAGUS
Family: Liliaceae 天门冬
Asparagus cochinchinensis
shiny asparagus

A profusely branched scrambling plant with many backward-pointing spines, the asparagus is native to southern China and Japan. True leaves are scale-like and inconspicuous. The foliage is represented by small, green, leaf-like branches. Flowers are white and solitary or in pairs. Fruits are white berries, each with a rounded, black seed.

Parts used:
roots: expel phlegm from the respiratory passages; increase flow of urine; tonic for females; treat hacking cough, spitting of blood, fever, constipation arising after a fever

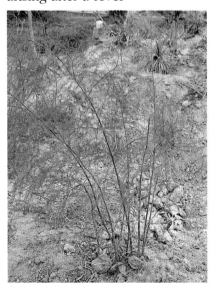
Asparagus

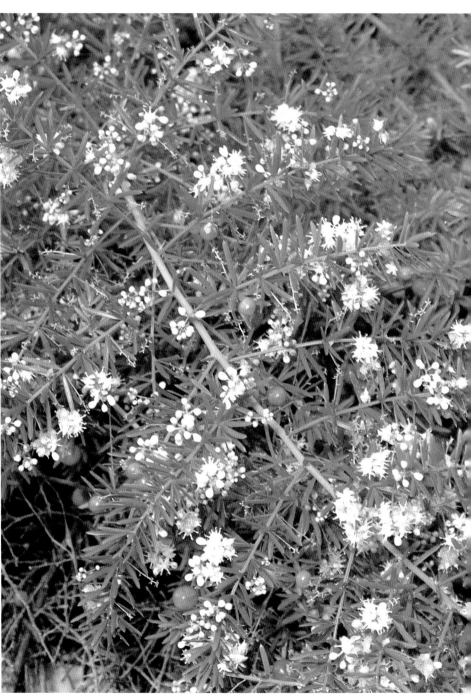
Asparagus

34

ASTER
Family: Compositae
Aster tataricus 紫菀
Tartarian aster

The name *Aster* comes from the Latin word, *aster*, for "star". The plant, native to northern China, Siberia and Japan, is a tall shrub covered with minute bristles and leaves of varying shapes and sizes. Flower heads are in large, loose bunches, the central flowers being yellow and the marginal ones blue-purple.

Parts used:
underground rootstock: purgative; treats colds, coughs with excessive sputum or with blood, whooping cough, painful menstruation

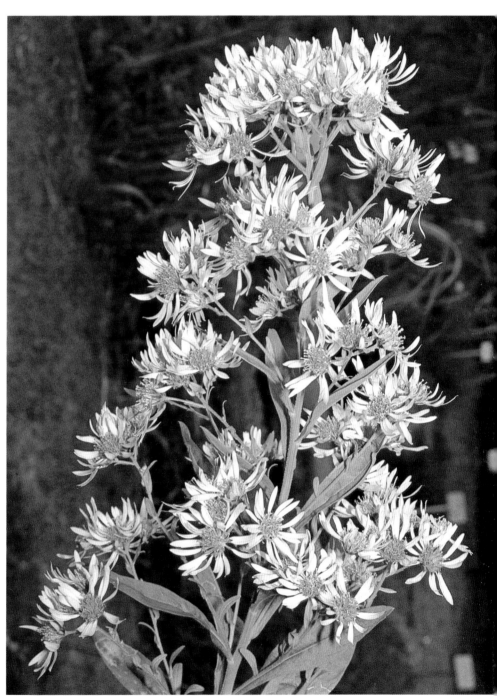

Aster tataricus

35

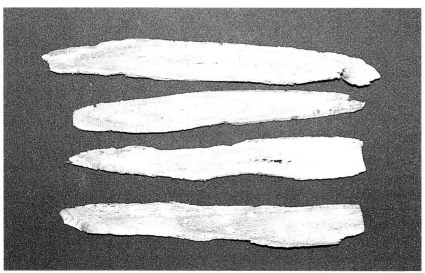

Astragalus membranaceus

ASTRAGALUS
Family: Leguminosae
Astragalus membranaceus 黄耆
milk vetch

The milk vetch is a temperate herb of the northern hemisphere. The dried roots are jet black on the surface; the inner tissues of a white outer ring enclose a pale yellow inner core. They are used in Chinese medicine, sometimes after roasting with honey.

Parts used:
roots: treat common cold, arthritic pains and numbness, loss of appetite, weakness, abnormally small amount of urine discharge, sweating at night, numbness of the muscles, boils, diarrhoea, asthma, nervousness

ATRACTYLIS
Family: Compositae
Atractylis

Atractylis is a herb found in the region from Manchuria and Korea to northern and eastern China, and Japan.

Atractylis ovata 白术
Parts used:
roots: treat indigestion, skin problems, diarrhoea, fever, stomach disorders, night blindness

Atractylis macrocephala 白术
Parts used:
roots: sedative; mild purgative; treat loss of appetite, indigestion, chronic bronchitis, cough, anaemia during pregnancy

AVERRHOA
Family: Oxalidaceae
Averrhoa carambola 阳桃
starfruit

The generic name of the starfruit, *Averrhoa*, honours the Arabian physician, Averrhoes (1149–1217). The common name comes from the fruit, which is star-shaped in cross-section. The plant is native to the Malayan region, now widely distributed throughout the tropics. It is planted for the juicy fruits which are used as a vegetable or fresh fruit. Quality of the fruits is very variable: some are extremely sweet while others very sour.

Parts used:
fruits: increase flow of urine; treat wounds; arrest bleeding

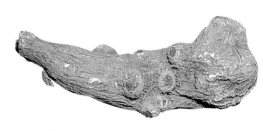

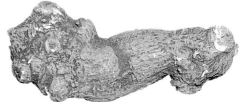

Atractylis macrocephala

36

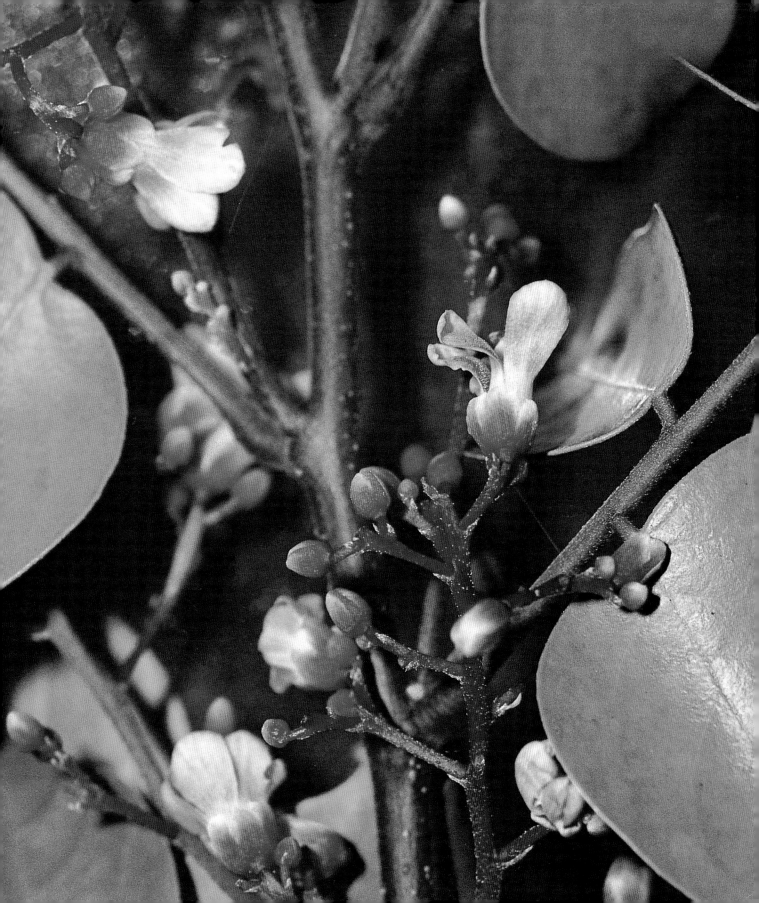

Bambusa

BAECKEA
Family: Myrtaceae
Baeckea frutescens 岗松
baeckea

This is a small, evergreen tree of Australasian origin, often seen by the sea or on mountain tops. Leaves are needle-like and aromatic. The dried leaves are placed among clothing to keep insects away.

Parts used:
leaves: treat sunstroke, fever

BAMBUSA
Family: Gramineae
Bambusa arundinacea
giant thorny bamboo

Bamboo is a Malay name and *Bambusa* is the Latinized version. Bamboos are easily recognized by their slender to thick, tall and straight stems which are hollow in the centre except at the nodes, which are marked by rings along the entire length.

The giant thorny bamboo, a native Indian plant, was introduced widely in the tropics and the subtropics. It has golden-yellow stems, growing to a height of 35 m, and lower branchlets which are thorny, thus the common name. In India the plants usually die after flowering at about the age of 30 years. This plant provides the

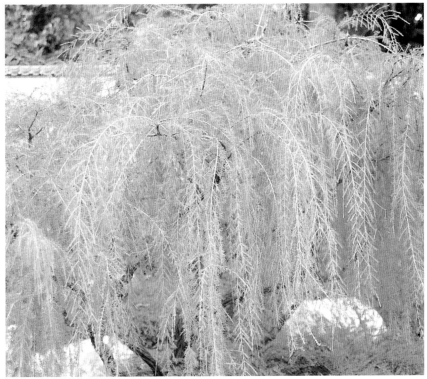

Baeckea frutescens

best bamboo for building structures.

Parts used:
stem sap, unfolded leaves: treat fever, rheumatism

BELAMCANDA
Family: Iridaceae
Belamcanda chinensis 射干
black-berry lily
leopard flower

The plant is a herb, native to China and Japan. The flowers are showy and deep orange in colour, with red dots. As the flower gets old, it twists spirally. The name black-berry lily comes from the fruit: once it splits open, the large, round, shiny black seeds appear, in clusters.

Parts used:
underground stem: cools the body system; treats tonsilitis, laryngitis, coughs, asthma, stomachache, swollen liver and spleen, painful urination, gonorrhoea, malaria, breast cancer

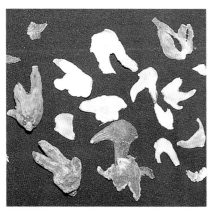

Bletilla striata

BENINCASA
Family: Cucurbitaceae
Benincasa hispida 冬瓜
Chinese preserving melon
white gourd
wax gourd

The plant is an annual, that is, it lasts only a year. It is native to Southeast Asia but now grown all over Asia. The hairy stem runs along the ground, bearing heart-shaped to kidney-shaped leaves. Fruits are nearly round to oblong, hairy and waxy-white, with white flesh and many white seeds. The young gourds are eaten as a vegetable while the old ones are used for making sweet pickles and preserves. The seeds are eaten fried. Young leaves and flower buds are eaten as vegetables.

Parts used:
seeds, fruits: mild laxative; tonic; reduce fever; treat piles, intestinal inflammation, diabetes, urinary and kidney diseases, gonorrhoea
rind: reduces fever

BLETILLA
Family: Orchidaceae
Bletilla striata 白及
bletilla

This is a ground orchid with purple flowers, native to China and Japan.

Parts used:
stem: tonic for the lungs; treats coughs, chest pain, blood in the sputum, abscesses, external bleeding, tuberculosis patients who vomit blood, swellings, dry and cracked skin, burns and scalds

BRASSICA
Family: Cruciferae
Brassica
mustard

Brassica is the classical name for cabbage. The plants are herbs or small shrubs, native to north temperate parts of the eastern hemisphere, with many growing as weeds. Four species are recorded in use by Chinese herbalists.

Brassica juncea 芥菜
Indian mustard
mustard greens

Parts used:
seeds: treat colds, stomach problems, abscesses, rheumatism, lumbago, skin eruptions, ulcers
leaves: treat inflammation of the bladder

Brassica cernua
Parts used:
seeds: treat pain in nerves, arthritis, pneumonia

Brassica napiformis 蔓菁
Parts used:
seeds: treat diabetes

Brassica oleracea var. *gongylodes* 甘蓝
Parts used:
leaves: tonic; aid to digestion

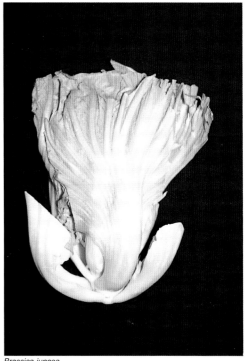

Brassica juncea

40

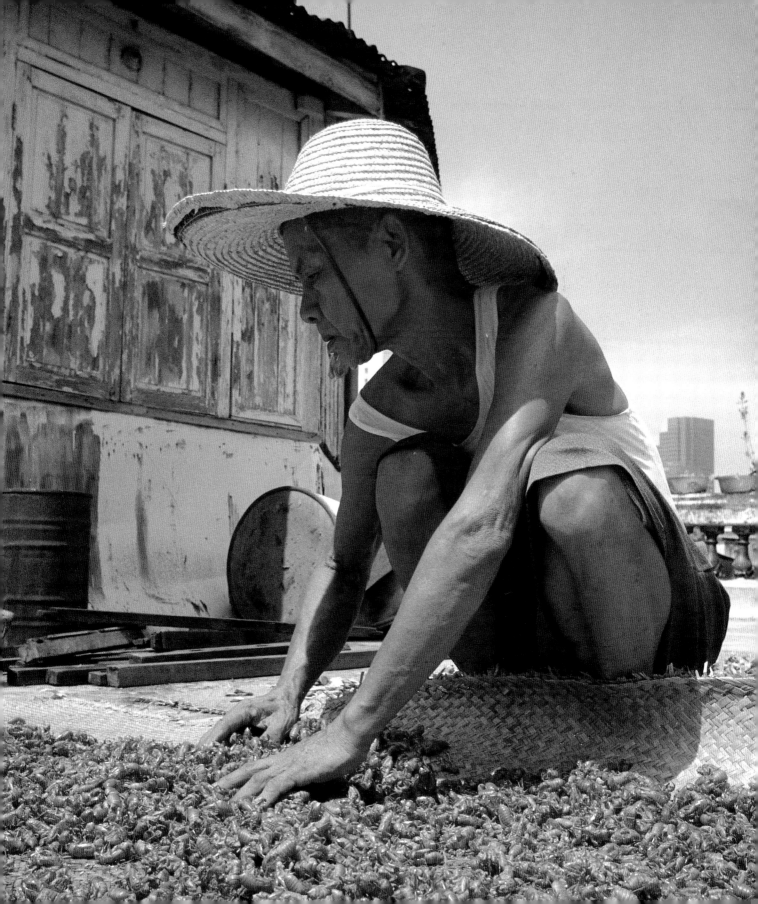

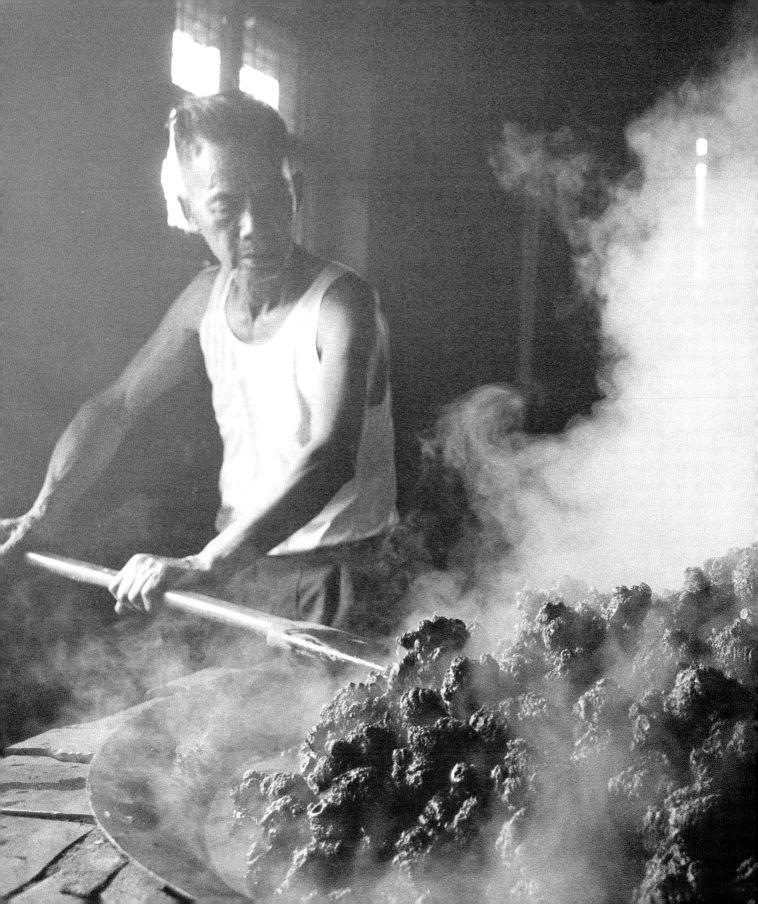

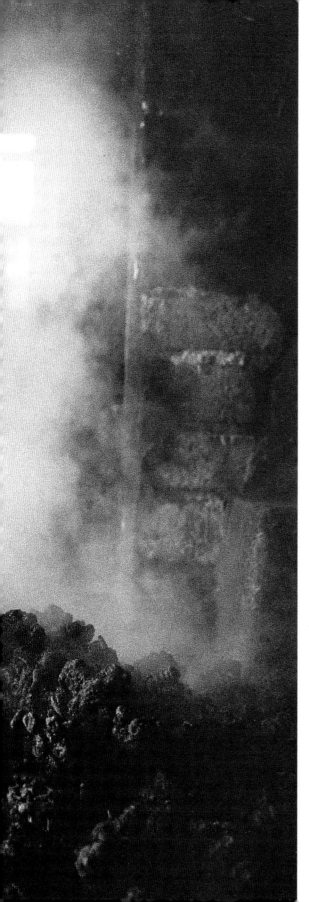

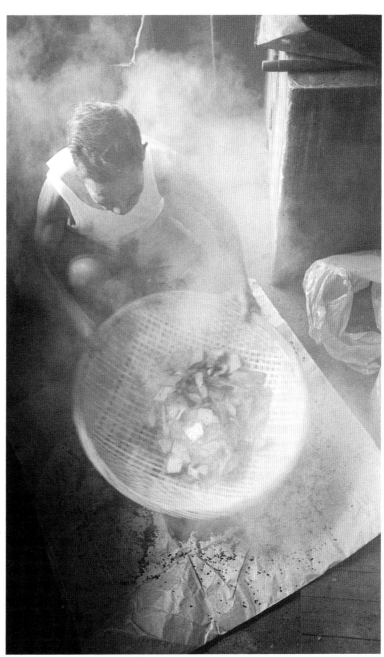

Frying is another way of drying out herbs.

Sometimes herbs are soaked and boiled in solutions to add to their potency.

43

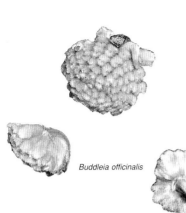

Buddleia officinalis

BRUCEA
Family: Simaroubaceae
Brucea javanica 鸦胆子
brucea

Brucea is a small shrub, native
to China, East Indies and the
Malay Archipelago. The seeds,
which contain an alkaloid and
taste bitterish, have been in use
in Chinese medicine for more
than two centuries.

Parts used:
seeds: mild laxative; tonic; treat
diarrhoea, piles, chronic
dysentery, amoebic dysentery

BUDDLEIA
Family: Loganiaceae
Buddleia
butterfly bush

Buddleia comes from the name
of an English botanist, Adam
Buddle (1660–1715). The plant
is a hairy shrub, native to
western China. The flower buds
are medicinal, containing the
alkaloid, buddlein.

Buddleia officinalis 密蒙花
Parts used:
flowers, leaves: treat night
blindness, cataract, eyestrain

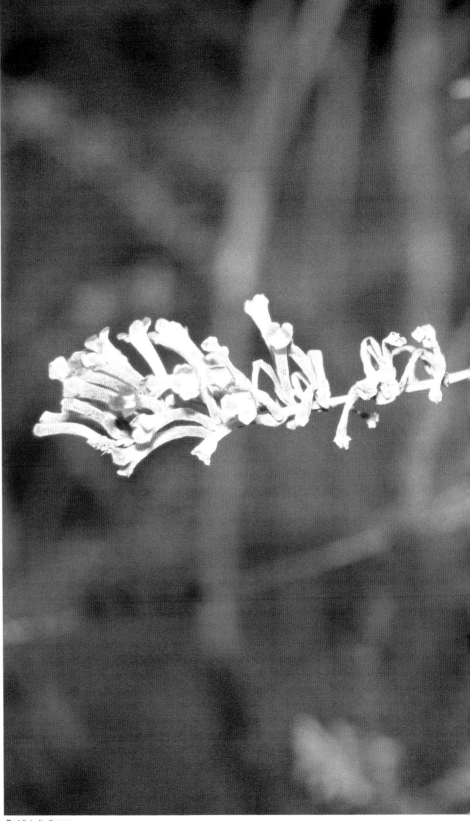

Buddleia lindleyana

44

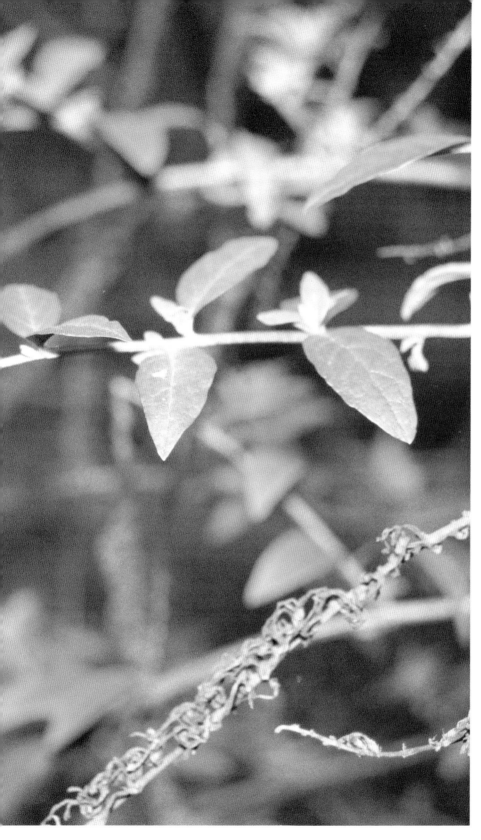

Buddleia lindleyana 醉鱼草
This is a poisonous plant which is used to stupefy fish and as an insecticide.

Parts used:
roots: treat asthma, coughing with blood

BUPLEURUM
Family: Umbelliferae
Bupleurum falcatum var. *scorzonerifolium* 狭叶柴胡
hare's ear

The plant is a slender herb with longish simple leaves and yellow flowers, native to northern China, northern Asia and Europe.

Parts used:
roots, plant: treat fever, deafness, dizziness, indigestion, common cold, gas in the system, rheumatism, jaundice, prolonged diarrhoea, malaria, inflammation of the liver and abdomen, irregular and absence of or painful menstruation

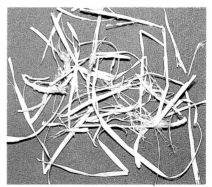

Bupleurum falcatum

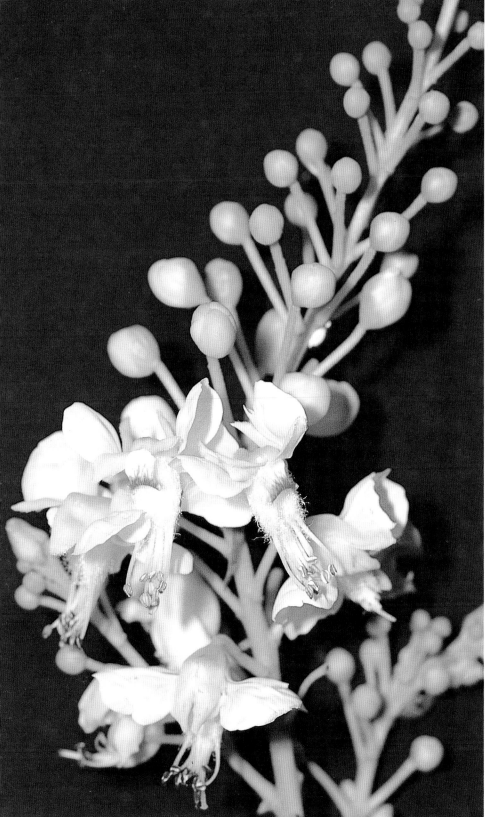

CAESALPINIA
FAMILY: Leguminosae
Caesalpinia sappan 苏木
sappan tree
brazilwood

The sappan tree is a small, prickly, evergreen tree, native to India and the Malay Peninsula. The heartwood yields a red dye which was popular before the introduction of synthetic aniline dyes. Chinese medicine values the heartwood, which is red. A decoction of this wood is used, from China to Indonesia and the Philippines, to treat problems related to blood.

Parts used:
heartwood: given to women after labour as a tonic; treats bruises, coughing and spitting of blood, bleeding during and after childbirth, purging of blood, excessive flow during menstruation

CAMELLIA
FAMILY: Theaceae
Camellia
camellia

Named after George Joseph Camellus, a Moravian Jesuit who travelled in Asia in the 17th century, camellias are shrubs and small trees native to East Asia.

Camellia japonica 山茶
common camellia

The common camellia is native to Japan and China. It is a popular ornament and has long been planted in the Far East for its beautiful flowers, but now extensively grown in warm temperate countries throughout the world. The flowers are unique in form and colour with spots often occurring under cultivation. They are large and showy, single or double, and of various colours from red to pink, or white or even variegated. There are more than 2000 named cultivars.

Because of the red colour of the flowers, the dried petals, flower buds and flowers are used in treatments associated with bleeding.

Parts used:
flowers: treat nose bleed, bleeding of the uterus, coughing of blood, burns and scalds

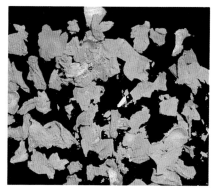
Camellia japonica

Camellia sinensis 茶
tea

The tea plant is actually a tree capable of growing to a height of 15 m. However, under cultivation it is intentionally kept under 2 m to enable pickers to harvest the young leaves. Flowers are white and fragrant, appearing singly or in small groups of three to four. A native of Southeast and East Asia, the tea plant is widely grown in warm temperate regions of East and South Asia and at higher altitudes in Southeast Asia. The young leaves are harvested and processed into tea, the world's most important caffein-based beverage.

Tea has been known in China for 3000 years. From here it was introduced to Europe in the 16th century but it was only in the 18th century that tea drinking finally caught on. There are two main types of tea: green tea, where the leaves are steam-dried without being allowed to ferment, and black tea, where the leaves are fermented and dried.

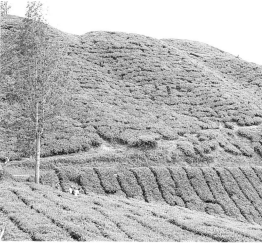
Camellia sinensis

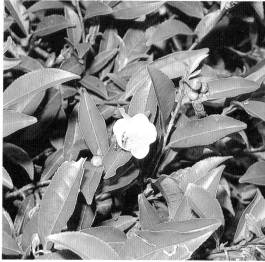
Camellia sinensis

Parts used:
leaves: stimulate the central nervous system; tonic for the heart; increase flow of urine

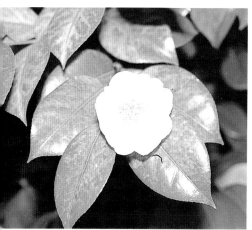
Camellia japonica

CAMPSIS
FAMILY: Bignoniaceae
Campsis grandiflora 紫葳
Chinese trumpet creeper
Chinese trumpet flower

This is a woody vine which climbs by means of aerial rootlets. The leaves are compound and in opposite pairs and the flowers are large, scarlet and in terminal bunches. The generic name, *Campsis*, is Greek for curve, and refers to the curved stamens.

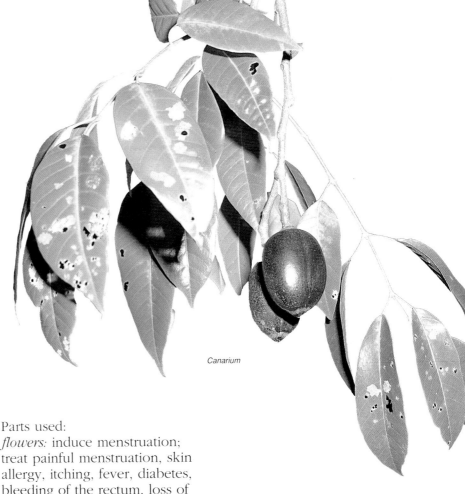

Canarium

Parts used:
flowers: induce menstruation; treat painful menstruation, skin allergy, itching, fever, diabetes, bleeding of the rectum, loss of appetite in children
roots: treat rheumatoid arthritis, paralysis of single limb or group of muscles

CANARIUM
FAMILY: Burseraceae
Canarium album 橄榄
canarium
kenari-nut tree

The kenari-nut tree, a native of Indo-China and South China, is valued for the oily kernel of the fruit, which is used in confectionery. The oil obtained from the kernel is used for cooking. The fresh and preserved fruits of *C. album*, looking very much like olives and known as *buah canna*, are sold in local shops. The powdered seed is believed to dissolve fish bones swallowed accidentally, while juice from the kernel is reputed to soften bones lodged in the throat.

Parts used:
fruits: antidote for poisoning resulting from eating poisonous fish; treat sore throat, diarrhoea
powdered seed: treat general inflammation

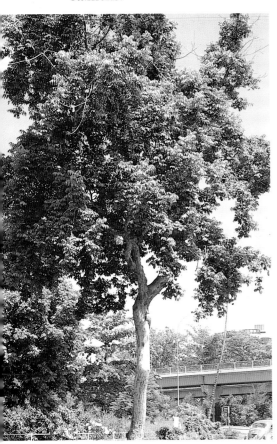

Canarium

CANNABIS
FAMILY: Cannabaceae

Cannabis sativa 大麻
hemp
marijuana
ganja
hashish

The herb is strong-smelling and covered with sticky hairs. It stands about 1 to 5 m high with the help of its woody, angular and hollow stem. Lower leaves are in opposites while upper ones are alternately arranged. The leaf blade appears like the palm of a hand, with 3 to 10 finger-like lobes. The leaf edge is toothed, appearing like the edge of a saw. Male flowers are greenish and in clusters, arising from the axils of leaves of the male plant. Female flowers are also greenish, but the clusters are terminal. The male plant dies soon after the last flower opens while the female plant continues living until the flowers become fruits and the fruits in turn mature. Fruits are smooth and shiny, and brownish in colour. The female plant is generally larger than the male. Hemp is thought to have originated in Asia Minor, from where it has spread to many areas in tropical Asia and America as well as many temperate regions. In many countries it is illegal to grow it.

The plant is grown for the fibres, used to make ropes; the male plant is said to give finer fibres. The fruits yield hemp-seed oil, used in the manufacture of varnish and soft soap. The seeds make excellent bird feed. The plant is also the source of three types of narcotics. From the dried leaves and flowering shoots of the male and female plants, hashish is produced. Ganja comes from the dried unfertilized female flowers of certain cultivars grown in India and from leafless twigs. The third type of narcotic is charas, the crude resin collected by rubbing the shoots with hands or beating them with a cloth. The active property of these drugs is a resin from the glandular hairs on the various parts of the plant. In the United States the dried top of the plant and leaves, known as marihuana or marijuana, are rolled into cigarettes and smoked. All the different narcotics are used as a stimulant, producing a state of euphoria which can lead, at high dosages, to mental confusion with illusions and hallucinations. However, the effect of the drug varies from individual to individual.

This plant has been associated with man for at least 10,000 years. According to Indian legend it was the gift of the gods to mankind, to enable man to achieve courage and heightened sexual desires

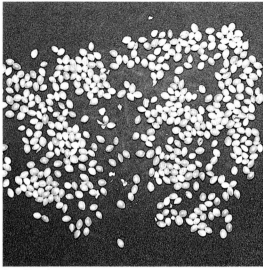

Cannabis sativa

through it. A Mahayana Buddhist tradition maintains that during the six steps of asceticism leading to his enlightenment, Buddha lived on one hemp seed a day. It has been in use in various traditional medicines since time immemorial, although its early usage must have been tied up with its euphoric and hallucinogenic properties.

Parts used:
ripe fruit, seeds: constipation following fever or labour
seeds: tonic; narcotic and pain killer; increase menstrual flow; increase flow of urine; expel intestinal worms; treat ulcers, wounds, skin eruptions
whole plant: treats indigestion, cancer, ulcers, migraine, rheumatism

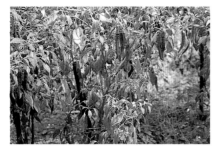

Capsicum annum

CAPSICUM
FAMILY: Solanaceae
Capsicum annuum 辣椒
chilli
pepper

The plant is a tropical American herb widely grown for the fruit, used as a spice or eaten as a vegetable. Fruits vary greatly in size and shape, from long and narrow to almost spherical, as many cultivars exist. They also vary in degree of pungency.

Parts used:
leaves: treat toothache
fruits: stimulate gastric activities; quicken blood circulation

CARICA
FAMILY: Caricaceae
Carica papaya 番木瓜
papaya
papaw
pawpaw

The origin of the plant is not known although it is believed that it came from southern

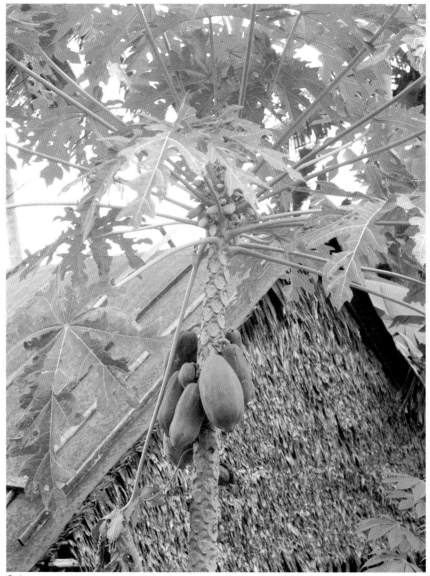

Carica papaya

Mexico and Costa Rica. It is now widely grown in most tropical and subtropical countries. The fruits are eaten fresh or canned as fruit salad together with other fruits. Unripe fruits can be eaten cooked or made into pickles. From the dried latex of unripe fruits papain is produced. It is used as a meat tenderizer, in the manufacture of chewing gum and cosmetics, and in the tanning of leather.

Parts used:
dried fruit pulp: reduce swelling and inflammation of the feet
fresh leaves: treat ulcers, swellings, boils and wounds
latex: expels intestinal worms; treats enlarged spleens; removes skin blemishes, freckles, warts and corns

CARTHAMUS
FAMILY: Compositae
Carthamus tinctorius 红花
false saffron
bastard saffron
safflower

Since antiquity, the flowers of false saffron have been a source of a delicate rose and rich scarlet colours. They have also been used in the production of the cosmetic rouge. A water-soluble yellow dye and an alcohol-soluble red dye, saffron carmine, can be extracted from the plant. The generic name is Arabic in origin, alluding to the colour obtained from the flowers. The plant is a stiff herb, about 1 m high, and thought to originate from Eurasia. It has never been found in the wild, being found in cultivation mainly in the Old World. The plant is also grown for the edible oil, obtained from the

seeds, and used as a basic ingredient in the production of certain margarines and cooking oil. The tender shoots are edible.

The plant is another excellent example of the doctrine of signatures. The red flowers are used mainly to treat problems related to blood. Extracts of the plant have been shown to have purgative properties as well as the ability to relax smooth muscles.

Parts used:
flowers: stimulate blood circulation; induce menstruation; treat painful menstruation, coughing of blood, internal bleeding, difficulty in discharging after-birth; prescribed to women carrying a dead foetus

CASSIA
FAMILY: Leguminosae
Cassia tora 决明
sicklepod
sickle senna

This is a small herb, native to southern China, Indochina, India, Japan, the Philippines and Indonesia. The flowers are showy and yellow, and generally grouped one to three in the leaf axils. Fruits are elongated pods, four-angled, and up to 12 cm long and 4 mm wide.

Parts used:
seeds: treat earache, dizziness, inflammation of the eyes, abnormal sensitivity of the eyes to light, constipation, herpes, sores and skin diseases, conjunctivitis

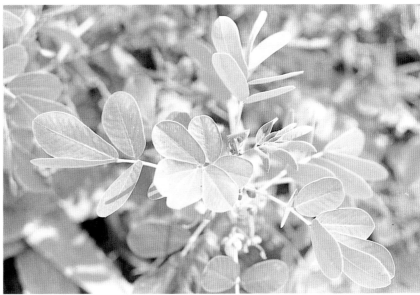
Cassia tora

51

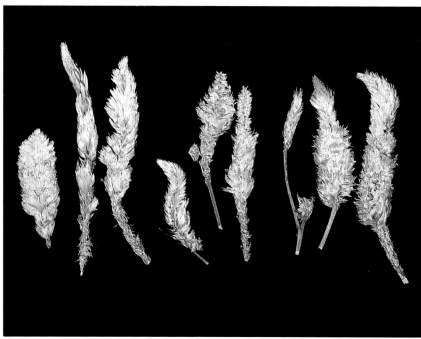

Celosia argentea

CELOSIA
FAMILY: Amarantaceae
Celosia
wool flower

The name *Celosia* is from the Greek *kelos*, "burned", alluding to the colour and appearance of the flowering branch of some species. *Celosia argentea* is a weed of Asian origin, now found in many tropical countries. The flowers are small and not individually showy, but obvious in the dense clusters, looking silvery white, thus the common name, wool flower.

Celosia cristata, cultivated as an ornament, has enlarged and

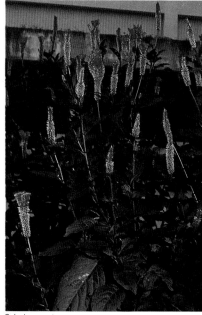

Celosia argentea

variously crested, plumed or feathered flowering terminal stems and branches, which are coloured yellow, purple or various shades of red. Its flowers are red. In Chinese medicine the usage of the two plants is the same, although the red-flowered one is generally preferred. This can be traced to the influence of the doctrine of signatures in which red flowers are appropriate in uses connected with the discharge of blood.

The plants were eaten by prisoners of war in Thailand during the Second World War to safeguard themselves against beriberi and pellagra, a disease caused by the absence of nicotinic acid in their diet. The plants have also been used as an aphrodisiac, and to treat cancer.

Celosia argentea 青葙
Celosia cristata 鸡冠花
cockscomb
Parts used:
whole plant: treats dysentery, coughing, spitting of blood, excessive discharge of blood during menstruation, absence of menstruation, bleeding of the intestines and lungs
seeds: treat "blurred eyes", inflammation of the eyes, abnormal sensitivity to light, headache; expel intestinal worms
leaf stalks: treat sores, wounds, boils, swellings

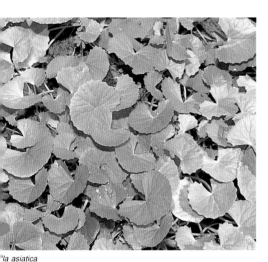

la asiatica

CENTELLA
FAMILY: Umbelliferae
Centella asiatica 积雪草
Asian pennywort
Indian pennywort

This is a common weed found in grassy areas all over the tropics. The plant has a thin creeping stem bearing, at intervals, bunches of rounded, heart-shaped leaves on a long stalk. Flowers are white, small and inconspicuous and fruits similarly small, elliptical, flattened and strongly ribbed. The plant is sometimes collected as a vegetable but most of the time it is used medicinally.

Parts used:
whole plant: stimulates appetite; aids digestion; treats bowel complaints in children, sores, ulcers and skin problems

CHAENOMELES
FAMILY: Rosaceae
Chaenomeles speciosa 宣木瓜
Japanese quince

Chaenomeles comes from the Greek words *chaino* and *meles*, meaning "split" and "apple" respectively, an allusion to the false belief that the fruit is split. These plants are deciduous shrubs of East Asia. Native to China, they are attractive and popular in Japan as ornaments, whether in its natural form or cultivated as bonsai. The fruits, roundish to pear-shaped, are fragrant, and used in Chinese medicine.

Parts used:
fruit: tonic; sedative; treats pains in the joints, sunstroke, nausea, indigestion, colic, cholera, rheumatism, diarrhoea, muscle spasms

CHIMONANTHUS
FAMILY: Calycanthaceae
Chimonanthus praecox 蜡梅
wintersweet

Flowers often bloom in midwinter, hence its generic name, *Chimonanthus*, which means "winter flower" in Greek, and its common name wintersweet. The fragrant yellow flowers appear when the shrub is bare of leaves, and long before the new leaves appear. A deciduous shrub, wintersweet is native to China.

Parts used:
flowers: treat sore throat, burns

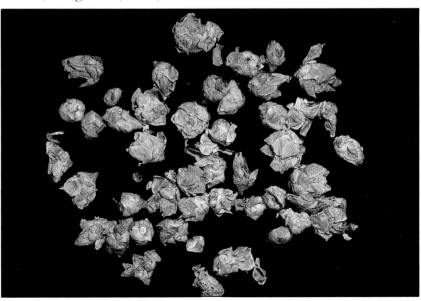

Chimonanthus praecox

53

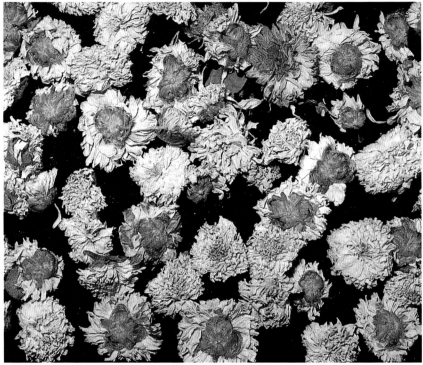

Chrysanthemum

CHRYSANTHEMUM
FAMILY: Compositae
Chrysanthemum
chrysanthemum

Chrysanthemum comes from the Greek *chyros*, meaning "golden" and *anthos*, "flower". The plant has been in cultivation for hundreds of years in the Far East. The chrysanthemum is to the East what the rose is to the West. A yellow chrysanthemum signifies dejection and slighted love; a white one truth; a red flower carries the sentiment of "I love you."

Chrysanthemum morifolium 菊
florist's chrysanthemum
The plant is of Chinese origin, believed to be a hybrid of a number of other species and subsequently selected by cultivators. It is a herb, bearing rather small flower heads in clusters. These heads are of various shapes and sizes as well as colours: from yellow, bronze, pink, many shades of red and purple to white. The leaves are lobed and strongly aromatic.

Florist's chrysanthemum is widely cultivated in China and Japan as ornaments and for the flower heads. The Chinese also cultivate certain cultivars for their edible petals, which add colour to salads. Flower heads are exported from the provinces of Shantou and Zhejiang in China. These heads are used to prepare chrysanthemum tea, known to the Chinese as *ju hua cha*. They are also used in the preparation of tonics and sedatives.

The plants are collected when in full bloom, dried in the shade, the flower heads removed and bleached in sulphur gas, and finally exposed to the air.

Parts used:
flowers: stimulate blood circulation; give clear vision; treat liver weakness, circulation problems, nervous problems, menstrual disorders, digestive problems, night blindness; improve potency

Chrysanthemum indicum 野菊
This is a much branched herb, native to Japan and China, and found in the wild. The flowers are yellow, with the heads about 3 cm across.

Parts used:
flowers: treat skin infections, high blood pressure
stem: treats skin infections

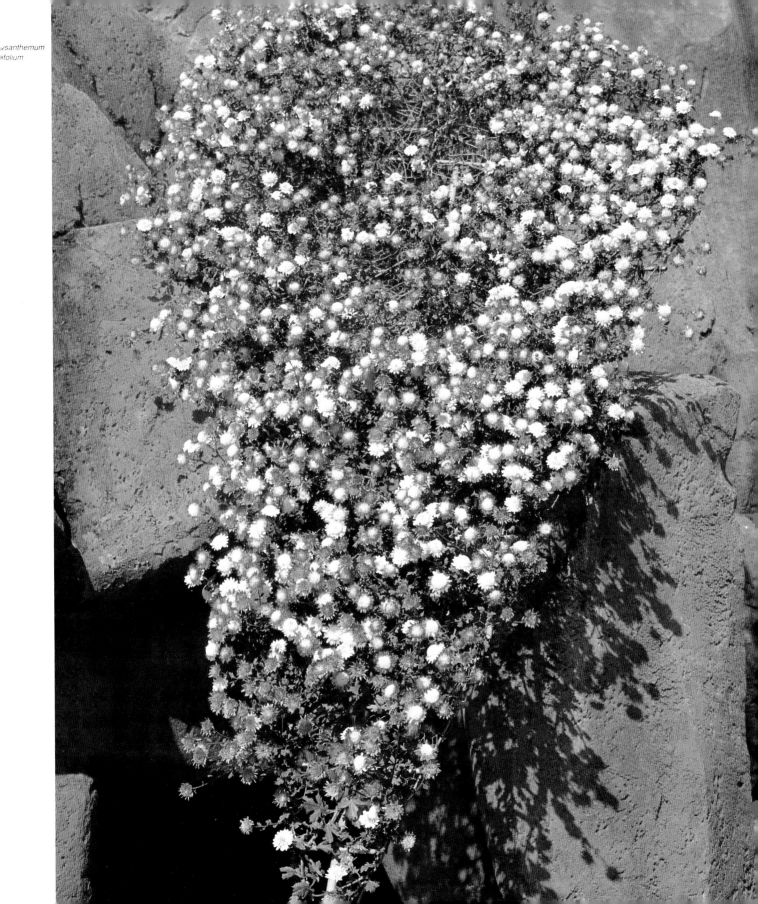

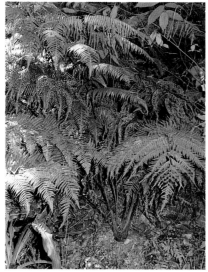
Cibotium barometz

CIBOTIUM
FAMILY: Dicksoniaceae
Cibotium barometz 金毛狗
Scythian lamb

This fern has a very short stem which is densely covered with brown hairs. It is a forest fern, native to China and the Malay Peninsula. The cut stems of certain Hawaiian species are used in horticulture as pots and planters.

The plant looks rather like a lamb: the stem portion forms the body and the leaf bases the legs, with the entire structure covered with golden hairs. This probably gave rise to the fable of the Scythian lamb, or vegetable lamb, which was said to grow on a stalk like a plant, and to devour other plants around it. The golden hairs have been on sale from a very long time ago for use to control bleeding. In Peninsular Malaysia the apical portion of the plant is commonly collected and sold as a charm. They are placed in pots of appropriate sizes and sold as "golden chickens", which are supposed to bring luck to the owner as well as ward off evil from the home.

Parts used:
stem: tonic for the liver and kidneys; purgative; digestive; promotes fertility; treats rheumatism, lumbago, bone diseases

CIMICIFUGA
FAMILY: Ranunculaceae
Cimicifuga foetida 升麻
bugbane

The generic name comes from the Latin words, *cimicis* and *fugio*, meaning "bug" and "to flee", as the plant was believed to have an insecticidal effect on bugs; thus also the common name, bugbane. The tall herb, reaching 2 m high, comes from the north temperate regions of southeastern Europe, Siberia and China.

Parts used:
roots: sedative; pain killer; treat measles, headache, diarrhoea

CINNAMOMUM
FAMILY: Lauraceae
Cinnamomum
cinnamomum

Cinnamomum is a group of aromatic trees and shrubs, native to the region stretching from East and Southeast Asia to Australia. The leaves are evergreen and in opposite pairs; each leaf has three prominent main veins and is leathery in texture. Several species are important sources of essential oil. The bark of *Cinnamomum zeylanicum* provides the spice cinnamon.

Cinnamomum camphora 樟
camphor tree
This is an evergreen tree, native to China, Taiwan and Japan. It is a popular ornamental tree of parks and waysides. The wood is used for camphor chests while the leaves, twigs and wood are distilled to produce camphor. Camphor may also be obtained from wounds made on the tree; it is valued by the Chinese for its many medicinal qualities. Camphor and camphorated oil are used externally to relieve pain, muscle aches and pains, and chest congestion, resulting from colds and bronchitis. Small pieces of camphor are placed in

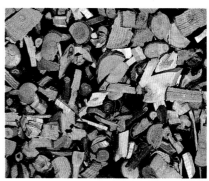
Cinnamomum cassia

boiling water and the vapour inhaled to clear colds and nasal congestion. The oil is rubbed on the chest and back as a treatment for colds.

Parts used:
camphor: treats colds, nasal congestion
camphorated oil: treats colds

Cinnamomum zeylanicum 锡兰肉桂
cinnamon

The cinnamon of commerce, which is used as a spice or condiment, for flavouring cakes and sweets, in curry powder, and in incense and perfumes, comes from the bark of this tree. A native of India, Sri Lanka and Peninsular Malaysia, it is now widely cultivated. In cultivation it is encouraged to branch from the base of the stem; each branch of three to five years' growth is cut off and the bark ripped off to be dried as the cinnamon of commerce.

Cinnamon oil, distilled from the dried green leaves, is used externally, in Chinese medicine, as an astringent, carminative and antiseptic. Consumed in light doses, it is believed to be a narcotic poison.

Parts used:
cinnamon oil: treats nausea, vomiting
bark: stimulates digestion, respiration and blood circulation; treats rheumatism, tuberculosis, headache

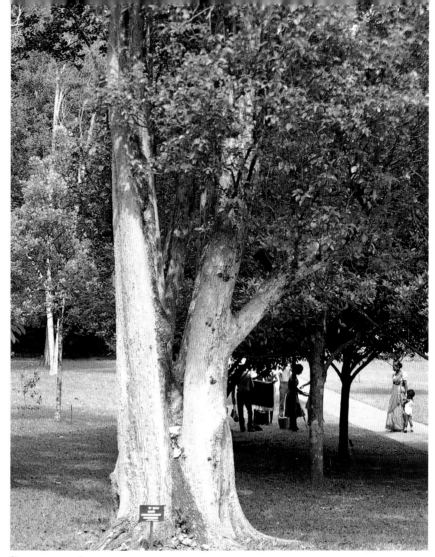

Cinnamomum camphora

Cinnamomum cassia 肉桂
Chinese cinnamon
cassia
cassia-bark tree

The tree is native to Burma but now cultivated in southern China and Indonesia. The bark was known in Europe in the 14th century as cinnamon and used then to produce incense, drugs and oils, as well as to mull wine, but not as a table spice. Cassia oil, obtained by the distillation of the unripe fruits, is used in chocolate and allied industries. The dried, unripe fruits, commonly known as cassia buds, are used as a spice.

Parts used:
bark, twigs: increase flow of urine; induce menstrual flow; treat painful menstruation, lumbago in old people, stomachache, indigestion, common cold, headache, fever
branches: induce sweating; promote blood circulation; treat fever, pain in the joints and abdomen

CITRUS
FAMILY: Rutaceae
Citrus
citrus

Citrus are evergreen spiny shrubs to small trees, native to South and Southeast Asia. The leaves are dotted with oil glands and aromatic when crushed. The fruits are thick skinned and roundish to oval in shape; several are important fruits of commerce such as the orange, mandarin, lemon and grapefruit.

Citrus medica 枸木缘
citron

This is a small, thorny tree, native to India but cultivated in Southeast Asia, the Mediterranean region, and the West Indies. Fruits are yellow, oblong, rough, and warty, with a thick rind and little pulp. The plant is grown for the thick rind, which is candied.

Parts used:
leaves, roots, fruit peel: treat lumbago

Citrus aurantium 酸橙
sour orange
bitter orange
seville orange

This is a spiny evergreen tree, native to southern Vietnam. The tree is now cultivated or naturalized in many tropical and subtropical countries. The leaf is simple, with the stalk typically

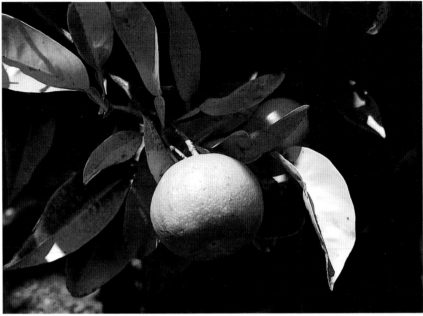

Citrus aurantium

winged. Flowers are white and very fragrant, while the fruits are globose, with a leathery skin which is dotted with oily glands, and orange to reddish when ripe. On ripening the segments separate, resulting in a hollow centre. The pulp is acidic and bitter, too bitter to be eaten as a fresh fruit. The cut fruit, like the crushed leaves, gives off a characteristic aromatic pungent odour.

The rind of the fruit is used to make marmalade and to flavour liqueurs. Various parts of the plant provide specific essence, very much in demand by the perfume industry for the making of *eau de cologne*. Neroli oil is obtained from the flowers, oil of *petit-grain* from the leaves and young shoots, and linolenic acid from the seeds.

Parts used:
ripe and unripe fruits: treat spleen and stomach ailments, chest congestion, abdominal pain, diarrhoea
seeds: treat pimples and freckles

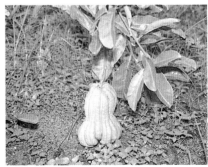

Citrus medica

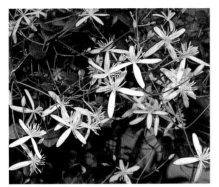
Clematis

CLEMATIS
FAMILY: Ranunculaceae
Clematis
clematis

Clematis comes from the Greek word *klematis*, meaning "climbing plant". Many species are prized as ornaments, planted as covers of fences and porches. Others are planted for their attractive flowers.

Clematis chinensis 威灵仙
virgin's bower
leather flower
vase vine
This is a climber with compound leaves of five leaflets and fragrant white flowers. It is native to China, Taiwan and Vietnam.

Parts used:
roots: laxative; antidote for alcohol poisoning; increase flow of urine; regulate menstruation; treat rheumatism, lumbago, backache, arthritis, jaundice

Clematis montana 绣球藤
This woody climber is native to the Himalayas and China. It has compound leaves with three toothed leaflets. The flowers are in clusters, fragrant, and white in colour, gradually turning pink with age.

Parts used:
stems: treat painful urination, excessive discharge of urine, insomnia, restlessness

CLERODENDRON
FAMILY: Verbenaceae
Clerodendron
glory-bower
Kashmir-bouquet
tubeflower

These are shrubs or trees, native to the tropics. The flowers are colourful – red, yellow, orange, blue or white. The generic name, *Clerodendron*, is Greek for "chance" and "tree"; of what significance this has, no one knows.

Clerodendron trichotomum 臭梧桐
This is an attractive and graceful ornamental shrub, with fragrant white flowers and bright blue fruits sitting on fleshy red bases. It originates from Japan.

Parts used:
leaves: treat hypertension, rheumatic pains, dermatitis

Clerodendron inerme 苦郎树
wild jasmine
Indian privet
This evergreen shrub is indigenous to the mangrove areas near Bombay. Flowers are small, white, and fragrant, with long, whiskery, purple stamens.

Parts used:
leaves: wash for skin diseases; treat beriberi

Clerodendron japonicum 赪桐
This attractive shrub, with red to scarlet flowers, is native to Japan and China.

Parts used:
leaves: treat gonorrhoea, nose bleed, bleeding of the bowels

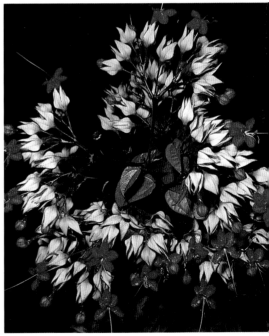
Clerodendron

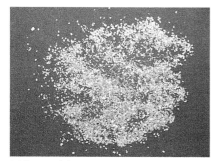

Cnidium monnieri

CNIDIUM
FAMILY: Umbelliferae
Cnidium monnieri 蛇床
cnidium

This herb is native to China, Siberia and eastern Europe. It has highly dissected compound leaves; small, white flowers in compact heads; and oval, brown, and slightly compressed, fruits. The seeds, grey-yellow and tasting bitter, are medicinal, and used as a stimulant, aphrodisiac, and sedative.

Parts used:
seeds: increase menstrual flow; treat rheumatism, kidney problems, wounds, yellow discharge from the vagina, piles, scabies

CODONOPSIS
FAMILY: Campanulaceae
Codonopsis pilosula 党参
bonnet bellflower

This plant is a twining herb, native to northeastern Asia. It has tuberous roots, and leaves

which are heart-shaped and strong-smelling when crushed. Flowers are pale green, tinged with purple at the top, solitary and on long stalks. They look like bells, thus the common name, and the generic name of *Codonopsis*, Greek for "bell-like". There is a belief that the roots have aphrodisiac properties, thus their widespread use as a substitute for the more expensive ginseng.

Parts used:
roots: tonic; preventive medicine for gonorrhoea; treat loss of appetite, loss of memory, asthma, weakness after a fever, insomnia, heart palpitation, blood pressure, diabetes, cancer of the breast, menstrual problems

Codonopsis tangshen, native to west China, is similarly used.

COIX
FAMILY: Gramineae
Coix lacryma-jobi 薏苡
Job's tears

The generic name of Job's tears, *Coix*, comes from the Greek *koix*, meaning "palm", a name given by Linnaeus, the Swedish botanist who established the binomial system of classification of plants. The specific name, *lacryma-jobi*, means "tears of Job", a fanciful allusion to the

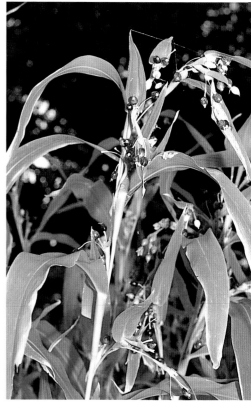

Coix lacryma-jobi

large tear-like sheaths enclosing the flowers. This stout and tufted grass, native to Southeast Asia, is popularly cultivated as an ornament and for the fruits, eaten as food in Southeast Asian countries or used as beads for necklaces and rosaries. The kernels are used medicinally in China, Japan, India and the Philippines. They are used as a diuretic, tonic, emollient and sedative, and to stimulate gastric activities and reduce fever.

Parts used:
kernels: treat lung and chest complaints, rheumatism, dropsy, gonorrhoea

COPTIS
FAMILY: Ranunculaceae
Coptis chinensis 黄连
goldthread

This is a herb, native to temperate China. The underground stem yields a yellow dye and is medicinal. It is sometimes used to induce the secretion of milk in women after childbirth.

Parts used:
underground stem: treats fever, vomiting, diarrhoea, nausea, bleeding, conjunctivitis

CORNUS
FAMILY: Cornaceae
Cornus officinalis 山茱萸
Japanese cornel
Japanese cornelian cherry

The generic name, *Cornus*, is from the Latin *cornu*, meaning "horn", a reference to the toughness of the wood. This is a small tree or shrub, with small, yellow flowers developing in early spring when the plant is bare of leaves. The plant comes from eastern China, Korea and Japan. In China the fruits are collected when they are purplered. They are soaked in brine to hasten subsequent drying as well as to preserve better. The medicinal properties of the fruits are supposed to improve with age. A quinol glucoside has been isolated from the plant and this could be the reason for the alleged effectiveness in the treatment of excessive discharge of urine.

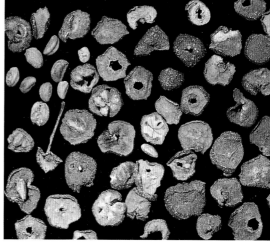

Crataegus pinnatifida

Parts used:
fruits: tonic; expel intestinal worms; treat lumbago, dizziness, backache, sweating at night, impotence, excessive discharge of urine, excessive menstruation, fever

CRATAEGUS
FAMILY: Rosaceae
Crataegus cuneata 野山楂
hawthorn
Crataegus pinnatifida 山楂
Chinese hill haw

The scientific name, *Crataegus*, comes from the Greek *kratos*, meaning "strength", alluding to the hardness of the wood. These plants are mostly thorny, deciduous shrubs or short trees, native to the north temperate zones.

Parts used:
ripe fruits: treat diarrhoea, dysentery, stomachache after birth

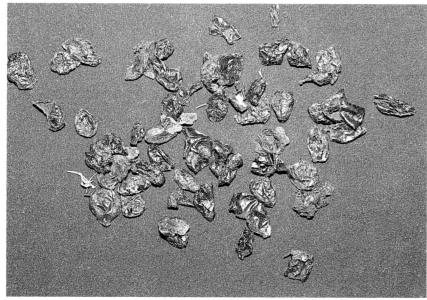

Cornus officinalis

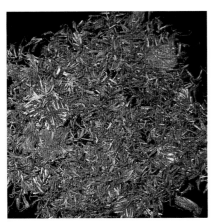

Crocus sativus

CROCUS
FAMILY: Iridaceae
Crocus sativus 番红花
saffron
saffron crocus

The generic name of saffron, *Crocus*, comes from the Greek word *krokos*, meaning "saffron". It is an autumn flowering herbaceous plant with grasslike leaves arising from the short stem, which is an extension of the bulb. Flowers are lilac, reddish-purple or white, large and fragrant, with yellow anthers and branched blood-red styles. It is the dried stigmas of the flowers that yield the saffron of commerce. About 4000 flowers provide about 30 g of the dye. Saffron is an important food colouring and flavouring, used also as a colouring material for medicines. Known only in cultivation, the plant is believed to have originated from Asia Minor. It has been used as a source of a yellow dye in the Mediterranean region and in the Near East since antiquity and is still cultivated on a large scale in southern France and Spain. A dental pain killer is obtained from the stigmas.

The stigmas are used medicinally by the Chinese. The flowers are collected in the early mornings and taken indoors where the stigmas are removed, and dried over a slow heat.

Parts used:
stigmas: enrich blood; help blood circulation; hasten eruption of measles; treat irregular menstruation, absence of menstruation, bleeding after labour, asthma, whooping cough, convulsions

CROTON
FAMILY: Euphorbiaceae
Croton tiglium 巴豆
croton

Croton is a small, evergreen tree, native to southwestern China, Burma, Laos, Vietnam, and Malaysia. The leaves have a rounded base and a pointed tip, and turn red just before they fall. The plant is cultivated for its seeds in India and Sri Lanka, from which is obtained croton oil, a very powerful purgative. A

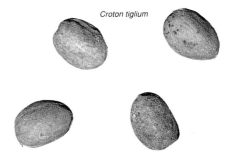

Croton tiglium

single drop of this oil is enough to cause diarrhoea, and higher doses can be fatal. Croton seeds were used in many European pharmacies up to the early 20th century. Analysis of the fruit oil has shown the presence of two active properties, one a purgative, the other an irritant. Seeds are poisonous but used medicinally in Chinese medicine as a violent purgative.

Parts used:
seeds: violent purgative

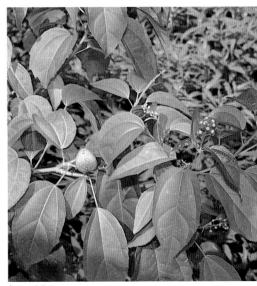

Croton tiglium

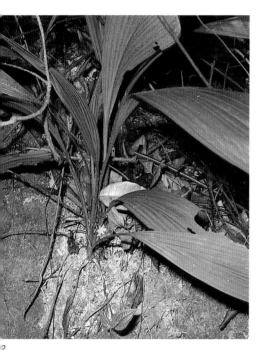

CURCULIGO
FAMILY: Hypoxidaceae
Curculigo orchioides 仙茅
curculigo

This is a herb with an underground stem, native to the tropics of the southern hemisphere – from India and the warmer parts of China, south to New Guinea. The leaves are long and pleated and the flowers are small and in dense bunches, borne near the ground.

Parts used:
underground stem: tonic; aphrodisiac; treats impotence, lumbago, pains in the joints

CURCUMA
FAMILY: Zingiberaceae
Curcuma domestica 姜黄
turmeric

Turmeric is a perennial herb, native to India but widely cultivated in the tropics. The plant has a stout underground stem which puts out shoots of about 1 m tall at intervals. Leaves are large, elongated and borne at the top of the non-woody stem. The pale yellow flowers are borne terminally on a stalk arising from the top of the stem. All parts of the plant are aromatic.

In Sanskrit "turmeric" means yellow, a sacred colour used by Hindus in body paintings during rites connected with birth, marriage and death. Up to today turmeric is an auspicious article in all Hindu religious observances. Turmeric powder was once used by the Hindus of India as a cosmetic.

It is widely cultivated in the tropics for the underground stem which may be dried or ground, and is used as a spice and a dye. It was an important dye in Asia as well as Europe prior to the discovery of aniline dyes.

Parts used:
underground stem: stimulates the production of red blood cells; dissolves blood clots; arrests bleedings; treats jaundice, irregular menstruation, stomach problems, pain in the abdomen, chest and back, diarrhoea, dysentery

Curcuma aromatica 郁金
wild turmeric
This plant is native to India.

Parts used:
underground stem: removes excessive gas from the system; increases menstrual flow; treats liver and stomach diseases, abdominal pains, convulsions, delirium, jaundice

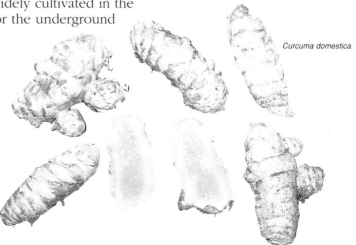

Curcuma domestica

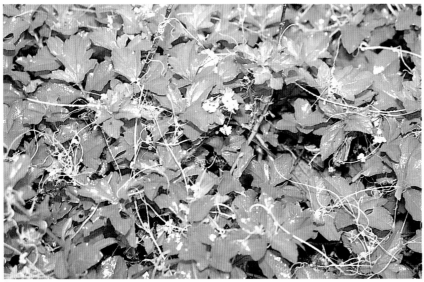
Cuscuta

CUSCUTA
FAMILY: Convolvulaceae
Cuscuta japonica 大菟丝子
dodder
lady's laces
bride's laces
devil's guts

The dodder is a leafless parasitic plant, native to China and Japan. Seeds give a threadlike stem which creeps along the ground until it comes into contact with a host plant. The slender, pale-green stem twines round and penetrates into the tissues of the host plant with the help of minute suckers, which siphon off nutrients. The rear portion then dies off and the plant becomes independent of the soil.

Parts used:
ripe seed, whole plant: treat lumbago, inflammation of prostate glands, nervous breakdown, dizziness, involuntary as well as excessive discharge of urine
seeds: treat premature ejaculation, impotence, yellowish discharge from the vagina

CYATHULA
FAMILY: Amarantaceae
Cyathula
hookweed

Hookweed is a straggling plant, so named because of the bundles of stiff, hooked hairs along the flowering spike. It is cosmopolitan in distribution and common in waste grounds.

Cyathula prostrata 杯苋
Parts used:
stem, leaves: mild laxative

Cyathula capitata 头花蒽草
Parts used:
roots: induce menstruation; treat rheumatism, arthritis, skin infection

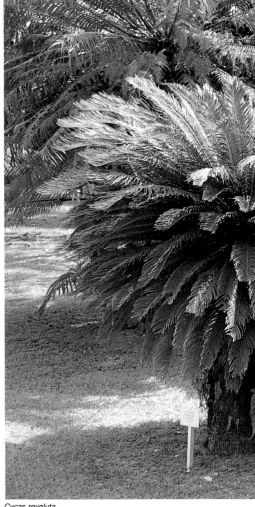
Cycas revoluta

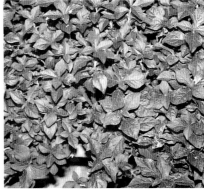
Cyathula prostrata

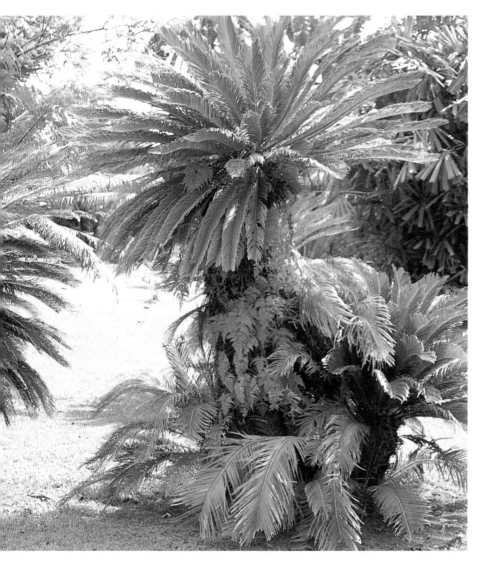

CYMBOPOGON
FAMILY: Gramineae
Cymbopogon citratus 香茅
lemon grass

This is a tufted grass with many stiff stems arising from short, underground rootstocks. Probably a native of southern India and Sri Lanka, it is widely grown in the tropics as a flavouring for food and for the essential oil it produces. Lemon grass oil is incorporated in soaps to provide a pleasant aroma and is used in perfumes. The Chinese boil the plant and drink the water to cure various ailments.

Parts used:
plant: treats coughs, colds, blood in sputum
roots: induce sweating; increase flow of urine

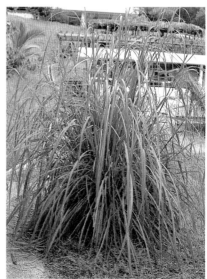

Cymbopogon citratus

CYCAS
FAMILY: Cycadaceae
Cycas revoluta 苏铁
Japanese fern palm
Japanese sago palm
sago palm

The generic name, *Cycas*, comes from the Greek name for a palm tree. A native of southern China and Japan, the tree has been exported and planted as ornaments in many countries. In Japan it is a favourite bonsai plant. The down on the young leaves and the woolly bracts bearing the female spores are used by the Chinese to treat wounds.

Parts used:
seeds: tonic; expel phlegm; increase menstrual flow; treat rheumatism

CYNANCHUM
FAMILY: Asclepiadaceae
Cynanchum
cynanchum

This is an upright and hairy alpine herb of northern China and Japan. The brownish red flowers are found in small clusters at the axils of leaves. The fragrant root is used in Chinese medicine.

Cynanchum atratum 直文白薇
Parts used:
roots: treat fever, coughs, blood in urine, inflammation of the urethra

Cynanchum glaucescens
芫花叶白前
Cynanchum stauntonii 柳叶白前
Parts used:
roots, stems: treat coughs, pneumonia, uneasy breathing, lung diseases

CYPERUS
FAMILY: Cyperaceae
Cyperus rotundus 莎草
nut grass

This is a troublesome weedy sedge with a creeping underground stem which bears oval tubers from which shoots develop. The plant has a main stem bearing long, narrow leaves and a central stalk ending in a terminal flowering branch. The flowering units are

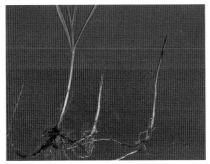
Cyperus rotundus

flattened; they bear small, three-angled nuts when mature. The tubers contain essential oils and are used to keep clothing fragrant. They can be burnt as a perfume or used as an insect repellent.

Parts used:
tubers: induce menstruation; treat painful menstruation, excessive menstrual bleeding, chest pains, stomachache, indigestion, nausea, dysentery, chills and colds, coughs, headaches

DATURA
FAMILY: Solanaceae
Datura metel 白曼陀罗
downy thorn apple
horn-of-plenty

The plant is a native of India, as reflected in the east Indian origin of both parts of the scientific name. However, there are others who believe that it originates from southwestern China. Whatever its origin, the plant has been naturalized in the tropics of both hemispheres and widely cultivated as a showy ornament. There are a number of cultivars which differ in the colour of the flowers. The flowers are up to 25 cm long and trumpet-shaped, developing into spiny, roundish fruits which split into a number of portions.

This is a poisonous plant with the leaves, fruits and seeds containing the largest amount of tropane alkaloids, the poisonous substances. The leaves and seeds of the plant are the source of an alkaloidal drug scopolamine, used in the prevention of travel sickness and in the production of sedative and truth serum (that is, it induces one to tell the truth).

It is sacred in China, the Buddhists believing that raindrops fell from heaven onto the plant when Buddha preached. In ancient Greece the priests of Apollo used the seeds to achieve a trance-like, prophetic state. Temple priests of the Incas used another species to sedate their patients prior to surgery. The seeds of some African *Datura* have been used in the initiation ceremony of African boys, to intoxicate and also for trials by ordeal.

Seeds of *Datura* have been used in criminal poisoning and to knock out a person prior to robbing him. In India, dancing girls used to drug wine with the

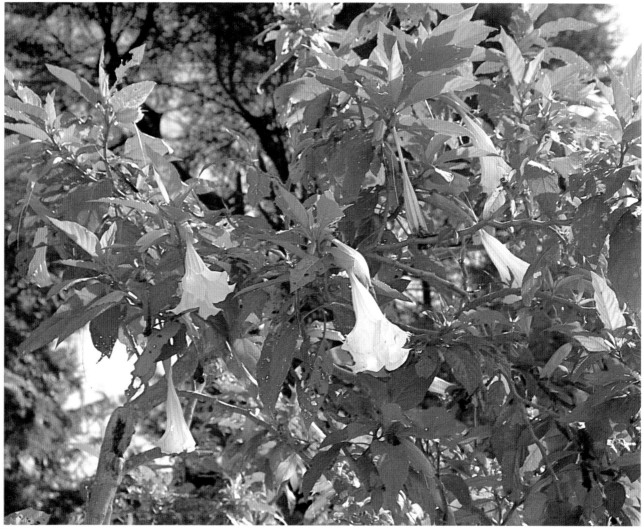

Datura

seeds and offer the drink to those they wish to rob or to extract answers to questions which would otherwise not be answered. Prostitutes similarly used the seeds to sedate their clients and rob them. There is also a report that women in the East breed beetles on the leaves of these plants and give the poisonous droppings to their unfaithful lovers. In Peninsular Malaysia robbers burn the seeds under the house of prospective victims and blow the smoke into the house; the fumes make the occupants unconscious and allow the robbers to ransack the house at leisure.

Parts used:
flowers: treat asthma, colds, nervous disorders, numbness, muscle pain

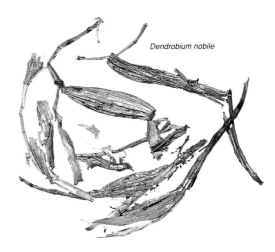
Dendrobium nobile

DENDROBIUM
FAMILY: Orchidaceae
Dendrobium
dendrobium

Dendrobium comes from the Greek compound *dendron* and *bios*, meaning "tree" and "life", referring to the growth of these orchids on the branches of trees. Many species are used in Chinese medicine, the most widely used being *Dendrobium nobile*.

Dendrobium nobile 金钗石斛
This is a perennial alpine orchid, native to the Himalayas, Burma and China. The plant has fleshy, yellowish and deeply furrowed stems which bear fleshy, oblong leaves and small, white or purple flowers, in small clusters. The dried stems are soft and yellowish, containing the chemical dendrobine.

Parts used:
stem: stimulates secretion of saliva in the treatment of fever and dehydration; sedative in arthritis

Dendrobium monile 细茎石斛
Parts used:
whole plant: tonic; promotes digestion; pain killer; sedative in the treatment of arthritis; treats impotence

Dendrobium hancockii 细叶石斛
Parts used:
stem: treats fever, cough, thirst

DESMODIUM
FAMILY: Leguminosae
Desmodium
desmodium

Desmodium is derived from the Greek word *desmos*, meaning "a chain", in reference to the jointed pods seen in certain species. These are climbers of worldwide distribution.

Desmodium triquetrum 葫芦茶
Parts used:
whole plant: expels intestinal worms; treats spasms in infants, indigestion, piles, abscesses

Desmodium pulchellum 牌钱树
Parts used:
whole plant: treats rheumatic fever, convulsions in infants, toothache; dissolves internal blood clots; aids digestion

Desmodium triflorum 三点金草
Parts used:
whole plant: treats dysentery

Desmodium styracifolium 金钱草
Parts used:
whole plant: treats colic

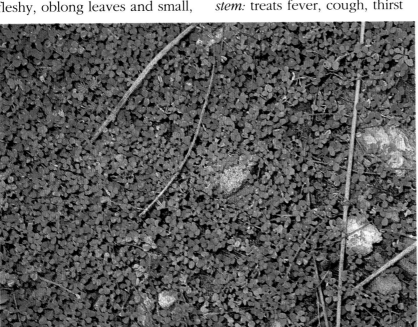
Desmodium triflorum

DIOSCOREA
FAMILY: Dioscoreaceae
Dioscorea
yam

The generic name, *Dioscorea*, is dedicated to Diosorides, Greek physician and naturalist (1st or 2nd century A.D.). The yam is a twining vine with underground tuberous roots. Many species, native to China, Japan and Korea, are actually grown and collected for use in Chinese medicine. Yams also have medicinal uses in many other Asian countries.

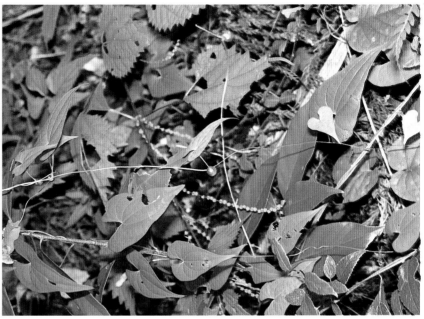
Dioscorea

Dioscorea opposita 薯蕷
Chinese yam
cinnamon vine

This yam is grown in China, Korea, Japan and Taiwan for its edible tuber which is spindle-shaped and may be as long as 1 m. During the mid-19th century when the potato was threatened by the blight in Europe, the Chinese yam was experimented with the view of using it as a substitute for the potato. The excessive mucilage present in the plant may be the reason for its effectiveness as a cough remedy, the mucilage having a soothing effect on the mucous membranes.

Parts used:
tubers: treat general weakness, diarrhoea, coughs, premature ejaculation, excessive discharge of urine, yellowish vaginal discharge

Dioscorea nipponica 穿龙薯蕷
Diosgenin, an active anti-inflammatory agent, has been isolated from this plant, thus supporting its use for rheumatoid arthritis.

Parts used:
tuber: treats rheumatoid arthritis

Dioscorea bulbifera 黄独
Parts used:
tubers: treat sore throat, boils, swellings, poisonous snake bites

Dioscorea tokoro 山萆薢
Parts used:
tubers: treat arthritis, rheumatism

Dioscorea japonica 日本薯蕷
Parts used:
tubers: treat indigestion, diarrhoea, dysentery

Dioscorea hispida 白薯莨
Parts used:
tubers: treat skin diseases

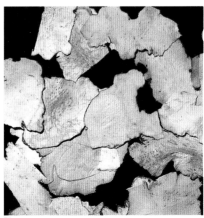
Dioscorea

DIOSPYROS
FAMILY: Ebenaceae
Diospyros kaki 柿
Japanese persimmon

The Japanese persimmon is a deciduous tree, native to Japan and China, where it is commonly planted for its edible fruits. The plant is now extensively grown in the Mediterranean countries. The brownish hairs covering the twigs and undersurface of the leaves are characteristic of the plant. The fruits are roundish, with an orange-yellow to reddish skin, orange pulp and flattened, elliptical seeds. The fresh as well as dried fruits are commonly sold in the market. Overripe fruit can be made into a jam. The pulp of the unripe fruit is used as the basis for face-packs in the cosmetic industry because of its firming qualities. In modern medicine the juice of the unripe fruit is used to treat high blood pressure, piles, typhus and typhoid. The fruit has laxative properties.

Parts used:
fruit: stimulates gastric activities; treats diarrhoea, piles
fruit juice: treats hypertension
fruit stalk: treats cough, hiccup

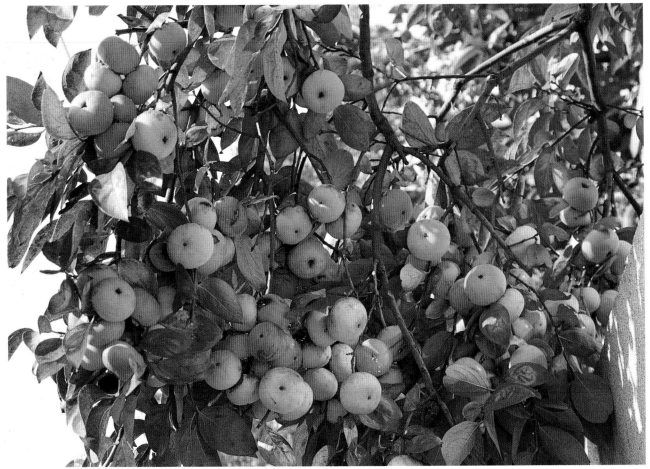

Diospyros kaki

DIPSACUS
FAMILY: Dipsacaceae
Dipsacus
teasel
Venus's basin

These are coarse, thorny herbs, native to Europe, western Asia and North Africa. The dried flower heads were once used in the domestic woollen industry for raising the nap of cloth. The leaf bases of some species join to form a hollow, which collects rainwater; thus the generic name from the Greek *dipsakos*, "thirst", and the common name, "Venus's basin".

Dipsacus asper 川续断
Dipsacus japonicus 续断
Parts used:
roots: treat lumbago, trauma as a result of a fall, rheumatic pain, excessive menstrual bleeding

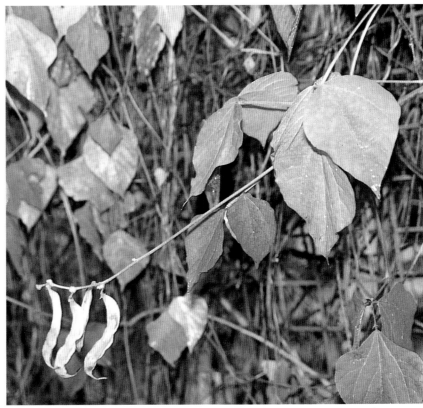
Dolichos lablab

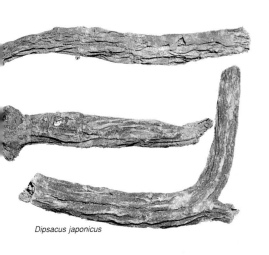
Dipsacus japonicus

DOLICHOS
FAMILY: Leguminosae
Dolichos lablab 扁豆
hyacinth bean
bovanist bean
lablab bean
seim bean
Indian bean
Egyptian bean

The generic name comes from an old Greek name of a bean. The plant is widely cultivated in the tropics and subtropics. It is probably of Asian origin and has been in culture in India for centuries. The young pods are eaten as a vegetable in India and elsewhere in the tropics. The ripe seeds are eaten as a split pulse in India.

Parts used:
flowers: treat dysentery when there is pus and bloody stools, inflammation of the uterus; increase menstrual flow
seeds: stimulate gastric activities; antidote against fish and vegetable poisoning; treat colic, cholera, diarrhoea, rheumatism, sunstroke

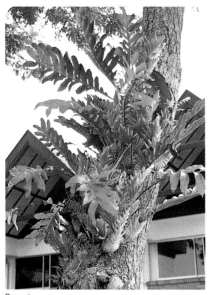

Drynaria

DRYNARIA
FAMILY: Polypodiaceae
Drynaria fortunei 槲蕨
oak-leaf fern

Oak-leaf fern is so named because its nest leaves resemble the leaves of the oak tree. The generic name, *Drynaria,* in fact, is Greek, meaning oak-like. This fern, which grows from the branches of trees, bears two types of leaves. The nest leaves, which grow close to the branches of the tree, are so called because they trap falling leaves which rot within the nest to provide nutrients to the roots. The normal leaves grow out from the creeping stem, which is protected by the nest leaves. These leaves bear the spore cases.

Parts used:
stem: controls bleeding; tonic for the kidneys; improves blood circulation; treats rheumatism, painful joints, fractures, gangrene, ulcers, wounds

DRYOBALANOPS
FAMILY: Dipterocarpaceae
Dryobalanops aromatica 龙脑香
kapur
Bornean camphor-tree

This is one of the tallest trees in the tropical forest, frequently growing to more than 70 m tall. Its distribution is confined to the Malay Peninsula, Java and Borneo. The tree was previously valued more for the camphor it produced than for the timber. The trees were felled and hacked into pieces for the camphor which was sold for medicinal purposes. The Chinese import the camphor into China and use it for medicinal purposes. The resin present in the tissues of the tree crystallizes within cavities of the trunk to become camphor.

Parts used:
camphor: tonic; aphrodisiac; treats chicken pox, poor eyesight, sore throat

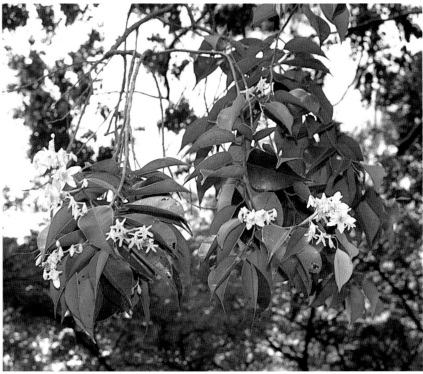

Dryobalanops aromatica

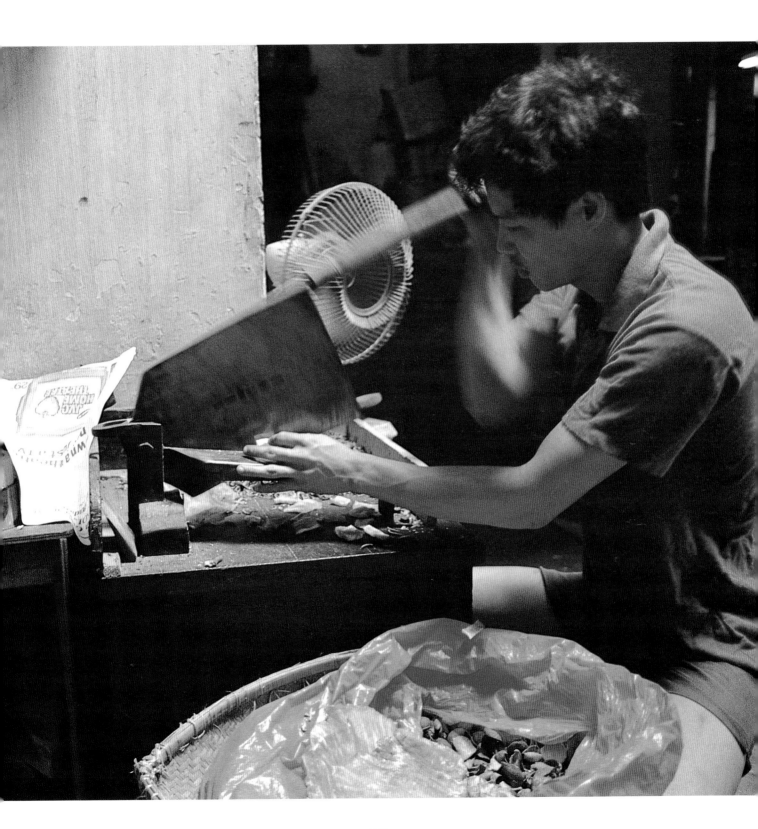

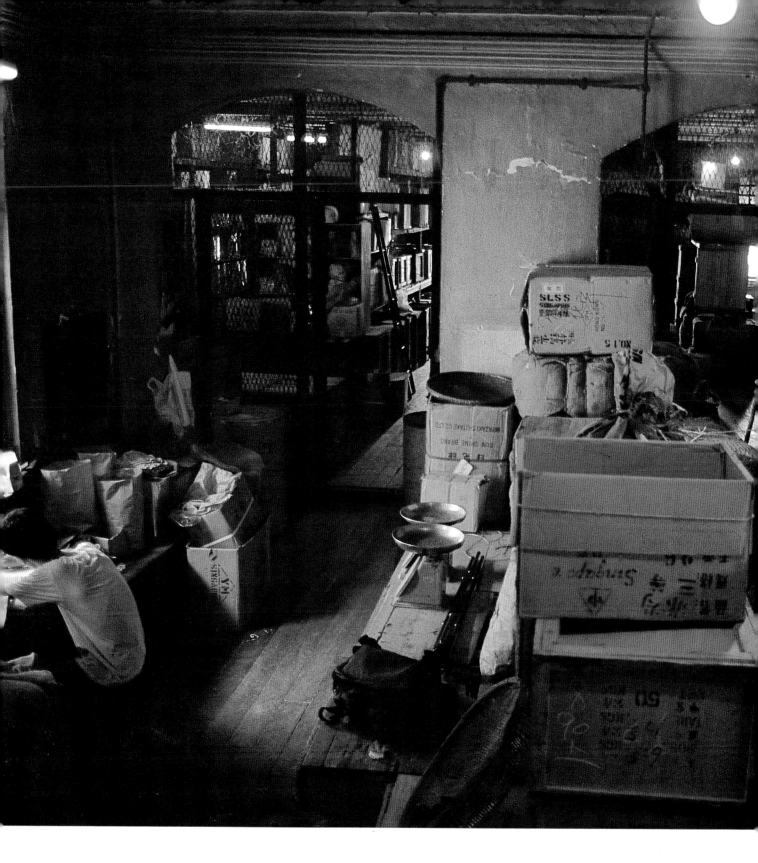

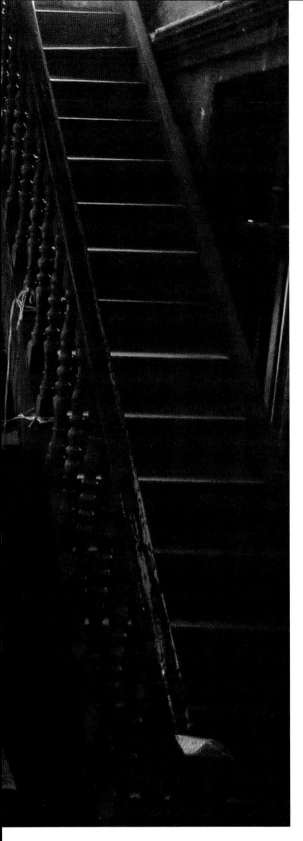

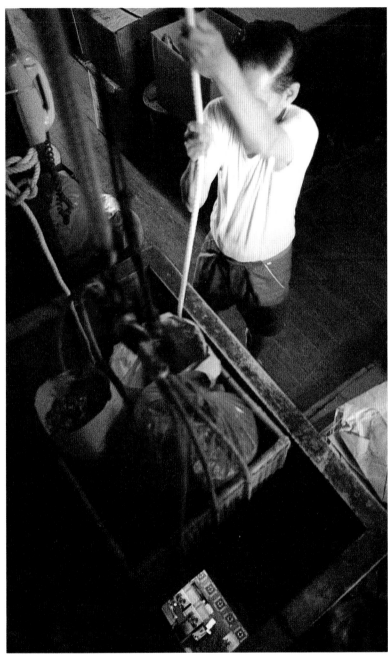

A dumb waiter of sorts, a basket on rope and
pulley, carries things from the warehouse floor
to the shop floor two storeys below.

On the cool and dimly lit warehouse floor of
the Eu Yan Sang medical hall herbs are
stored, in tins, urns or wooden crates.

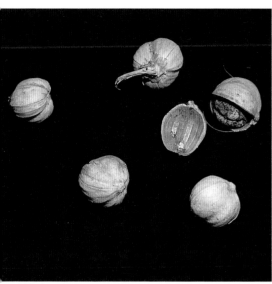

Elettaria cardamomum

ECLIPTA
FAMILY: Compositae
Eclipta prostrata 鱧肠
white heads

The plant is commonly known by the name of white heads because of its many stalked, white flowering heads arising from the leaf axils. It is a cosmopolitan weed, a herb found in China, Taiwan, Indochina, India, Japan, the Philippines and many other countries.

Parts used:
whole plant: treats dizziness, lumbago, blood in the vomit, lungs and urine, bleeding from cuts

ELETTARIA
FAMILY: Zingiberaceae
Elettaria cardamomum 小豆蔻
cardamom
Malabar cardamom
Ceylon cardamom
true cardamom

This herb, widely cultivated in Southeast Asia, is native to India and Sri Lanka. The plant bears flowers on a stalk arising from the rootstock. The attractive flowers have a white lip, with pink stripes. The fruits are thin-walled capsules holding aromatic seeds. These seeds are the true cardamom of commerce, used as a spice for seasoning, for medicine or as a masticatory. In the Middle East it is used to flavour coffee. It is also used in confectionery. An oil from the seeds is used in perfumery and for flavouring liqueurs and bitters. In the British and American pharmacopoeias it is used as an aromatic stimulant, carminative and a flavouring agent.

Parts used:
seeds: stimulate gastric activity; increase menstrual flow; treat premature ejaculation, involuntary discharge of urine, pain in the stomach
underground stem: tonic; laxative

ELSHOLTZIA
FAMILY: Labiatae
Elsholtzia splendens 海洲香薷
elsholtzia

The plant is named after the German physician and botanist, John Sigismund Elsholtz (1623–1688). This aromatic herb is cultivated in China; it is harvested when the seeds ripen. The stem is four-angled, with simple leaves attached in opposite pairs, each pair at right angle to the next. The flowers are small and purplish pink. All parts of the plant are covered with glandular hairs.

Parts used:
seeds: treat typhoid, colds, stomachache, vomiting

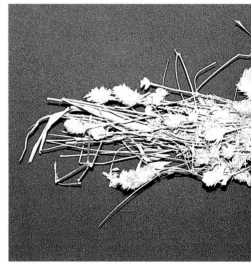

Elsholtzia splendens

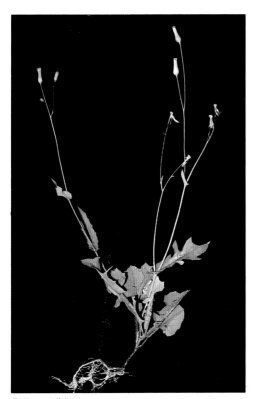

Emilia sonchifolia

EMILIA
FAMILY: Compositae
Emilia sonchifolia 一点红
Cupid's shaving brush

This is a weedy herb of the tropics. It has attractive pink flower heads which turn silky as the fruits develop. The plant is eaten as a salad in Indochina.

Parts used:
leaves: reduce fever; treat dysentery

EPHEDRA
FAMILY: Ephedraceae
Ephedra
joint fir

Joint fir is a much branched, shaggy shrub with slender green stems, found in dry or desert areas. The drug, ephedrine, used to treat coughs, asthma and hay fever, is obtained from the plant. This drug stimulates the heart and constricts blood vessels. It is also widely used in anaesthesia, and, because it may be taken orally, it is prescribed frequently for treatment of cold, sinusitis, hay fever and bronchial asthma. *Ma huang*, a species of ephedra, has been in use in China for more than 5000 years, for the treatment of asthma.

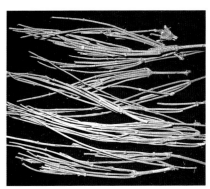

Ephedra sinica

Ephedra sinica 草麻黄
ma huang
Ephedra equisetina 木贼麻黄
Ephedra distachya 双穗麻黄
Parts used:
branches, roots: treat asthma, influenza, coughs, lung fever, chronic bronchitis, rheumatism, whooping cough, sweating in the night

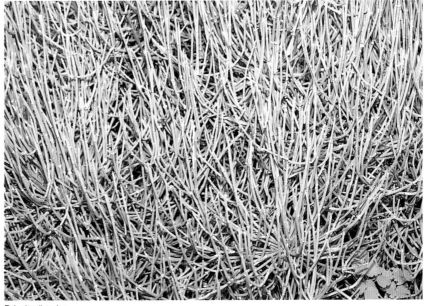

Ephedra distachya

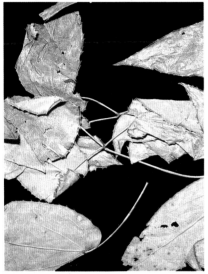
Epimedium

EPIMEDIUM
FAMILY: Berberidaceae
Epimedium

These are low herbs with underground stems, native to temperate Europe and Asia. They have small, compound leaves and equally small flowers.

Epimedium acuminatum 尖叶淫羊藿
Epimedium sagittatum 箭叶淫羊藿
Parts used:
whole plant: tonic; stimulates secretion of hormones; treats impotence, forgetfulness

EQUISETUM
FAMILY: Equisetaceae
Equisetum hyemale 木贼
common horsetail
common scouring rush

The family of treelike horsetails was once an important element of the earth's flora but it is now extinct, except for the herbaceous *Equisetum*. Many large fossils attest to the existence of the giant horsetails during the early years of the earth's history. Although closely related to the ferns, they differ from them, primarily in the pattern of organization of the plant body. Native to Eurasia and Pacific North America, it grows commonly in wet places.

It is an easily recognized herb, looking very much like a bunch of casuarina twigs, with its jointed stems and minute leaves found in whorls at the nodes. The stems are hollow and their surface grooved. They have a high silica content and are thus used for polishing tools and reeds of wind instruments. They have also been used as a crude sand paper and to clean copper objects. The plant is sometimes used by prospectors as an indicator of gold as it tends to accumulate the metal from the soil. It is an attractive ornamental plant and is often used in Japanese-style gardens.

Certain horsetails are poisonous, due to the presence

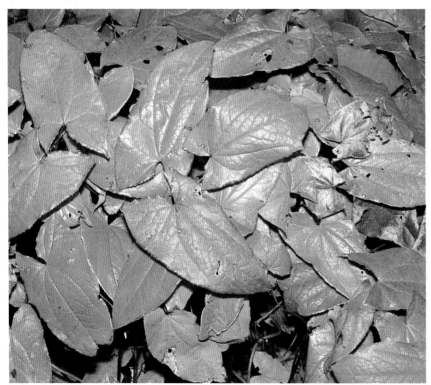
Epimedium sagittatum

of alkaloids in their tissues. Some contain the enzyme, thiaminase, which depletes vitamin B1 in grazing animals, resulting in nervous disorders. These plants contain several polyphenolic flavonoids which could exert a mild antibacterial effect. The medicinal usage of horsetail is seen in a number of cultures.

Parts used:
stem: retards bleeding; increases flow of urine; induces sweating during fever; treats dizziness, dysentery, piles, "cloudy eyes"

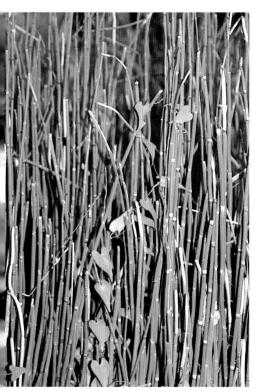

Equisetum hyemale

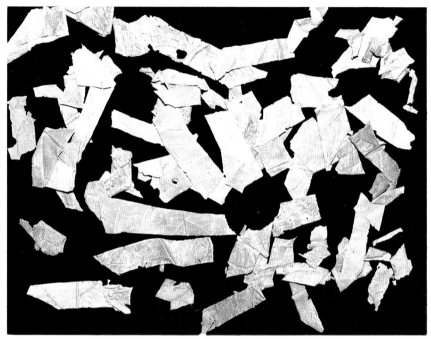

Eriobotrya japonica

ERIOBOTRYA
FAMILY: Rosaceae
Eriobotrya japonica 枇杷
loquat
Japanese medlar
Japanese plum

The plant has hairy flowering branches, thus the generic name, *Eriobotrya*, which is Greek for "woolly cluster". The evergreen tree grows to a height of about 7 m and develops a rounded crown. Flowers are white, occurring in rust-haired, terminal bunches. Fruits are fleshy, pear-shaped and yellowish. The plant is native to China and southern and central Japan where it is cultivated for the edible fruits. The effectiveness of the leaves in treating chronic bronchitis and coughs has been attributed to the saponin content. A decoction of flowers and leaves mixed with honey has been used to treat asthma and pain in the breast.

Parts used:
leaves: suppress coughs; expel mucus in the respiratory passages; treat stomachache, nausea, vomiting, cholera
bark: treats nausea, vomiting
fruits: treat nausea, cough
flowers: treat asthma, pain in the breast

79

ERIOCAULON
FAMILY: Eriocaulaceae
Eriocaulon buergerianum 谷精草
pipewort

Pipewort is a herb of swampy areas. The flower head resembles an eye, suggesting its use as a cure for sore and diseased eyes.

Parts used:
flower head with stalk: treats pain in the eyes, pain in the teeth, night blindness, cataract, fever, sore throat, headache

EUCOMMIA
FAMILY: Eucommiaceae
Eucommia ulmoides 杜仲
eucommia

The plant gets its generic name from the Greek words *eu* and *kommi*, meaning "true gum", alluding to the rubber content in the wood. This is a deciduous tree native to central China, in the provinces of Sichuan, Shaanxi, Hubei and Henan. The leaves are simple, elliptical to oblong-ovate, and elm-like. The latex and bark are used medicinally. The bark is peeled in spring and early

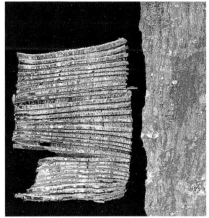
Eucommia ulmoides

summer, folded inwards, and tied with rice straws. They are then left for weeks until the inner surface becomes blackened, then untied and dried in the sun. In the preparation of the bark, the pieces are sliced into narrow strips but the presence of the dry latex, appearing like white threads, keep the strips together.

Parts used:
bark: tonic; treats backache, high blood pressure, threatened abortion, early stages of hypertension, impotence

EUONYMUS
FAMILY: Celastraceae
Euonymus
spindle tree

Many species of spindle trees are poisonous – the bark, leaves

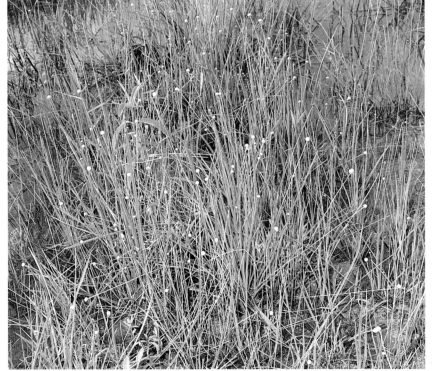
Eriocaulon

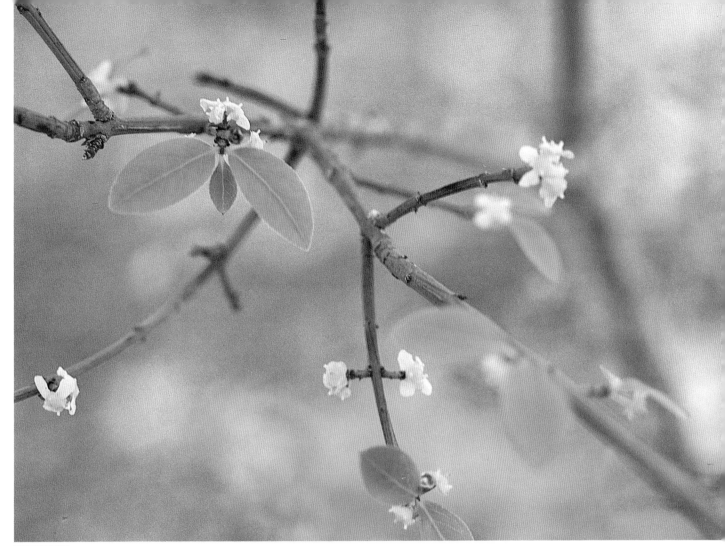

Euonymus alata

and fruits contain alkaloids and glycoside compounds. At one time the dried, powdered fruits of a spindle tree were used to treat lice and scabs and the oil from the seed was used externally for skin parasites and internally as a laxative.

Euonymus alata 卫矛
winged spindle tree

The tree is medium-sized and deciduous, with four-angled branches bearing two to four broad, corky wings. It is native to China and Japan. Flowers are small and greenish yellow, while fruits are purple, splitting at the base into four lobes to expose the brown seeds covered with an orange tissue. The plant has also been used as an insecticide.

Parts used:
corky wings of branches, branches: improve blood circulation; expel intestinal worms; treat pain after childbirth, irregular menstruation, malaria

Euonymus japonica 冬青卫矛
Japanese spindle tree

This is an evergreen shrub, sometimes growing into a small tree. The plant is native to Japan.

Parts used:
bark: tonic; aids difficult childbirth; treats rheumatism, night sweating

EUPATORIUM
FAMILY: Compositae
Eupatorium
boneset

Boneset is of cosmopolitan distribution, although found mainly in the tropics. The generic name *Eupatorium* is derived from that of an ancient king of Pontus, Mithridates Eupator, said by Pliny, the Roman naturalist, to have employed one of this group of plants in medicine. Many species are being used in herbal medicine throughout the world: from Europe to the Americas and Asia. In fact *Eupatorium* are some of the most important plants used in herbal medicine.

Eupatorium chinense 华泽兰
The plant is erect, with smallish flowering heads in dense bunches. It is native to Japan, Korea, Manchuria, China and the Philippines.

Parts used:
whole plant: treats colds, general weakness

Eupatorium fortunei 兰草
This species is found in China, Japan, and Indochina, where it is cultivated.

Part used:
whole plant: improves appetite; treats heat stroke with headache, fever, bad breath

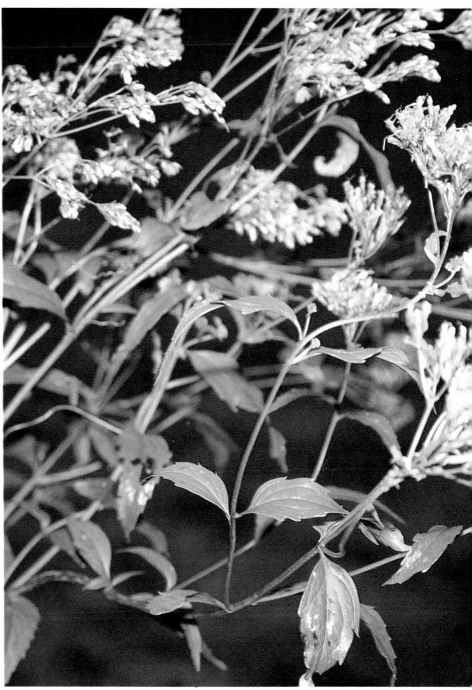

Eupatorium fortunei

82

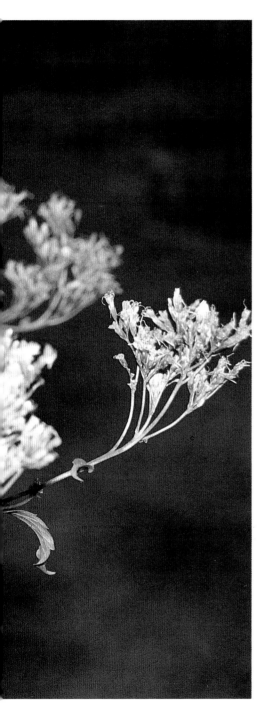

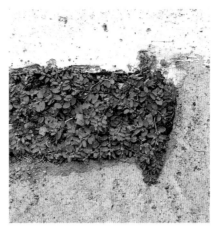

Euphorbia thymifolia

EUPHORBIA
FAMILY: Euphorbiaceae
Euphorbia thymifolia 千根草
thyme-leaved spurge

The name, spurge, originates from the Latin *expurgate*, "to cleanse", as certain species have purgative properties. This is a small, low-lying, tufted herbaceous plant, tinged reddish or purplish. It is a common weed of gardens and waste grounds.

Parts used:
whole plant: expels intestinal worms

EUPHORIA
FAMILY: Sapindaceae
Euphoria longan 龙眼
longan

The generic name, *Euphoria*, comes from the Greek words, *eu* and *phoros*, for "carries well", alluding to the attractive fruits. The longan is a well known fruit, native to India but widely cultivated in the Malay Archipelago and southern China. The tree is evergreen, with yellowish white, small flowers which are either unisexual or bisexual. These may be on the same tree or on different trees. Fruits are round and yellow-brown, with a juicy, white flesh surrounding a dark brown, shiny seed. In Chinese medicine, dried longan is considered to have warming and tonic properties.

Parts used:
flesh of fruit: contracts blood vessels; expels intestinal worms; treats nervous disorders
leaves: cool body system
flowers: treat kidney problems, yellowish discharge from vagina
roots: treat gonorrhoea, diabetes

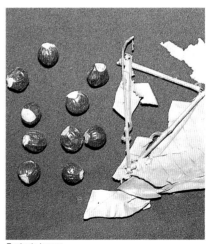

Euphoria longan

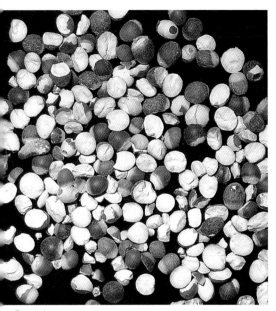

Euryale ferox

EURYALE
FAMILY: Nymphaeaceae
Euryale ferox 芡
prickly water lily

As the name implies, the plant has sepals which are reddish on the inner surface and green and prickly on the outer surface. Petals are purple. The leaves are large, up to 1 m or more across, and spiny-ribbed on the under surface. This aquatic plant is native to countries from China to northern India. In China, Japan and India, the plant is grown in still waters.

Parts used:
seeds: stimulate gastric activity; treat pain in the joints

FICUS
FAMILY: Moraceae
Ficus
figs

Figs are trees, shrubs or woody climbers native to the tropics, mainly of the Old World. All parts of the plant contain a milky sap which oozes out when the tissues are damaged. The leaves are simple and leathery or thick, and the flowers are confined inside oval to roundish figs, which have a small opening for the entry of fig wasps which help in pollination. Many species are stranglers, starting life on branches of trees, the roots going round the trunk to eventually strangle the host tree.

Ficus pumila 薜荔
creeping fig
climbing fig
creeping rubber plant
This is a vine, native to East Asia, from Japan to North Vietnam. It is commonly used to cover walls and other surfaces, as the many creeping roots arising from the stems cling on to such surfaces. The fruits are large figs, pear-shaped and yellowish. (Figs are false fruits, the inner wall of which contain the true fruits.) Planted over surfaces of walls, they need to be regularly pruned to maintain their attractive appearance. Also,

pruning keeps the plants vegetative, otherwise they bear figs, resulting in an untidy appearance.

Parts used:
stems, leaves: tonic for fever; treat wounds, boils, piles, sore throat, dysentery, rheumatism
fig: relieves hernia
roots: induce urination; treat inflammation of the bladder

Ficus retusa 榕树
Malayan banyan
Chinese banyan
Indian laurel
This is an evergreen tree, native to the region between India and New Guinea. The tree is recognized by the many aerial roots hanging from the branches and twigs, some developing into pillar roots once they touch the ground. It grows in swampy areas and, in the Malaysian region in particular, the trees are left alone when the forest is felled, as the local Chinese venerate them, making offerings and collecting the aerial roots for medicinal purposes.

Parts used:
figs: pain killer
leaves, buds: treat conjunctivitis
aerial roots: treat rheumatism, swollen feet, aching teeth

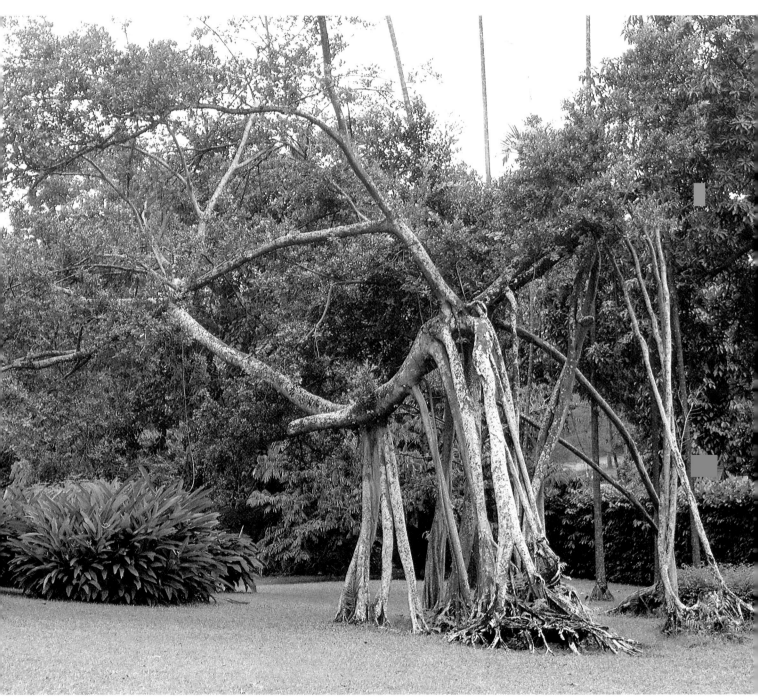

etusa

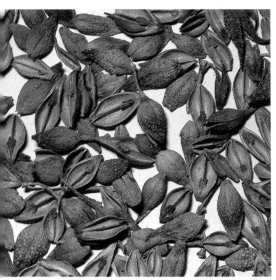
Forsythia suspensa

FIRMIANA
FAMILY: Sterculiaceae
Firmiana simplex 梧桐
Chinese parasol tree
Chinese bottle tree
phoenix tree

This tall, deciduous tree has leaves which have insecticidal properties. Native to East Asia, it is much planted as an ornament. It obtained its generic name, *Firmiana* from the Austrian Governor of Lombardy, Count K. J. von Firmiana (1716–1782).

Parts used:
seeds: treat abscesses in the mouth of children, skin problems
fruits: tonic
roots: reduce swellings

FORSYTHIA
FAMILY: Oleaceae
Forsythia suspensa 连翘
weeping golden-bell

The plant is named after the English horticulturist, William Forsyth (1737–1800). This medium-sized, deciduous shrub has slender, hollow branches which become pendulous, thus the weeping appearance. The small, golden-yellow flowers appear in profusion well before the leaves. This much planted ornament, especially as a spring-flowering shrub, is native to northern China. The dried, woody fruits, mainly without the seeds, are sold for medicinal use. The dried seeds are distinctly aromatic. The fruits contain saponins and the glucoside, phillyrin. The plant has a reputation for curing cancer and has been shown to have antitumour properties in experiments with animals.

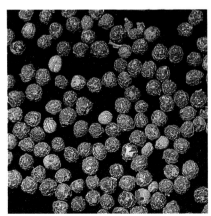
Firmiana simplex

Parts used:
fruits: alleviate inflammation; increase flow of urine; increase menstrual flow; expel pin worms; treat fever, headache, sore throat, tuberculosis of the lymphatic glands
leaves: treat skin problems, measles
leaf stalks: treat fever, ulcers, piles
roots: treat fever, colds, jaundice

FRITILLARIA
FAMILY: Liliaceae
Fritillaria
Fritillary

The generic name, *Fritillaria*, comes from the Latin, *fritillus*, "checker board", referring to the markings on floral parts of some species. The plant is a bulbous herb, native to western North America, Europe, Asia and North Africa.

Fritillaria cirrhose 卷叶贝母
Native to the Himalayas, its leaves are in opposite pairs or in whorls, with the upper leaves ending in tendril-like tips. Flowers are yellow-green and chequered with purple.

Parts used:
bulbs: treat chronic cough, chronic bronchitis, tuberculosis

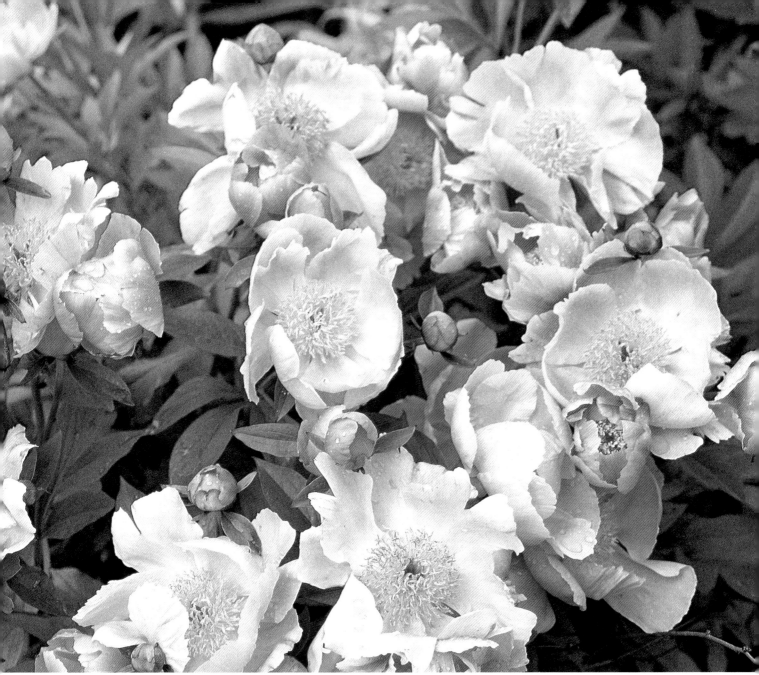

ia suffruticosa (see page 130)

Fritillaria verticillata var. *thunbergii*
浙贝母

The plant is native to China and Japan. In China it has been used to treat breast cancer while outside China it has been used for the treatment of other types of cancer. A number of steroidal alkaloids have been isolated, which can lower blood pressure, paralyze sensory nerves and respiration, cause vasoconstriction and cardiac and motor paralysis, and relax smooth muscles, in animals. These alkaloids are toxic, even lethal.

Parts used:
bulb: treats common cold, cough with phlegm, asthma, bronchitis, tuberculosis, painful menstruation, swelling, inflammation of the breast, stomachache

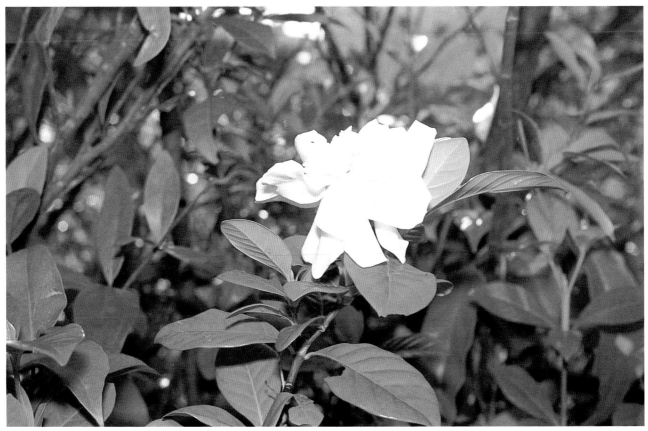

Gardenia jasminoides

GARDENIA
FAMILY: Rubiaceae

Gardenia jasminoides 山栀
common gardenia
cape jasmine

Gardenia is named after Alexander Garden (1730–1791), the physician from Charleston, United States, who was a correspondent of Linnaeus. Gardenias are popular garden plants, with large and attractive flowers. Native to China, it is also planted for cut flowers. The white flowers are highly fragrant, often growing in pairs.

Parts used:
fruits: treat vomiting of blood, bleeding, jaundice, acute gonorrhoea, sores, boils, abscesses, inflammation
seeds: treat jaundice, rheumatism, twisted muscles
flowers, roots: regulate flow of blood; control bleeding; increase menstrual flow

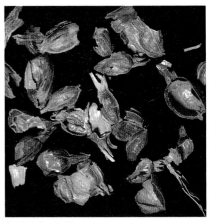

Gardenia jasminoides

GASTRODIA
FAMILY: Orchidaceae
Gastrodia elata 天麻

This orchid is native to East Asia. It lives on dead organic materials, being unable to manufacture its own food. The underground stems are dug out and used to treat various ailments.

Parts used:
underground stem: treats headache, dizziness, paralysis, lumbago, rheumatism

GENTIANA
FAMILY: Gentianaceae
Gentiana
gentian

Gentian is named after Gentius, King of Illyricum, a region roughly representing modern Yugoslavia; it is claimed that he discovered the medicinal properties of the plant about 2000 years ago. European herbalists used the powdered gentian roots in wine to treat snake bites, liver complaints, stomach pains, bruises, pain in the joints, and as a tonic. The plant is commonly used today as an antiseptic and a tonic. Almost all *Gentiana* species studied contain the alkaloid gentianine which has anti-inflammatory property when tested on animals. Thus the

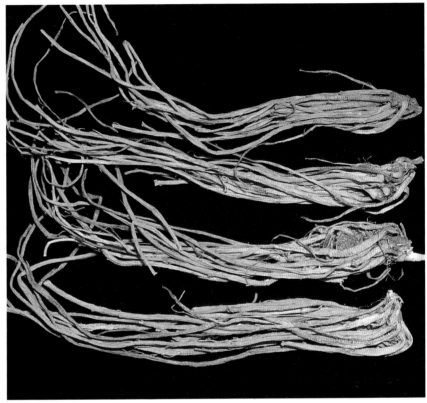

Gentiana scabra

rational basis for the treatment of rheumatoid arthritis.

Gentian is a tufted herb, mainly of temperate and arctic regions, or even montane areas of the tropics. The flowers are showy – white, yellow, blue, purple or red, and often spotted.

Gentiana macrophylla 大叶龙胆
This herb, from Siberia and northern China, has pale blue flowers. It contains bitter glucosides and is prescribed for various ailments.

Parts used:
roots: treat rheumatoid arthritis, fever, jaundice, convulsions, leprosy, tuberculosis, dysentery, piles

Gentiana scabra 龙胆
Japanese gentian
Gentiana triflora 三花龙胆
Parts used:
roots: treat inflammation of the eyes, rheumatoid arthritis, jaundice, fevers, common cold

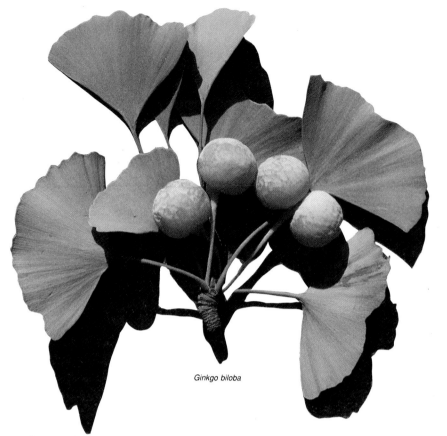

Ginkgo biloba

GINKGO
FAMILY: Ginkgoaceae
Ginkgo biloba 银杏
maidenhair tree
ginkgo

The plant is a very tall deciduous tree, native to East China but now probably extinct in the wild. However, it is frequently planted as a wayside or ornamental tree in temperate countries. The attractive feature of this tree is its fan-shaped leaves, frequently deeply notched in the middle, and borne on a long, slender stalk. The fruits are oval and yellowish, and give a smell like rancid butter when ripe. For this reason male trees are more desirable than female. On the other hand, female trees bear the fruits, the kernels of which are edible and much sought after in the East. The kernels, called ginkgo, are sold in China, Japan and various other countries in Southeast Asia, where they are considered a delicacy. A bonus in its consumption is that it is believed to aid digestion, besides being reputed to have the ability to expel intestinal worms. The leaves are placed between the pages of books, since ancient times in Japan, to protect them from insects. The seed coat has also been used as an insecticide.

Parts used:
young fruits: treat tuberculosis
fruit pulp: expels intestinal worms; treats coughs, asthma, bronchitis, kidney and bladder disorders, vaginal discharge, gonorrhoea

GLEDITSIA
FAMILY: Leguminosae
Gleditsia sinensis 皂荚
honey locust

The plant is named after Johann Gottlieb Gleditsch, director of the botanic gardens at Berlin (1714–1786). This is a medium-sized deciduous tree, native to China, and commonly planted along the wayside. The trunk and branches are armed with stout, sometimes branched, spines.

Parts used:
fruits, seeds: loosen mucus in the respiratory tracts; increase urine flow
leaves: treat wounds
bark, roots: expel intestinal worms; treat fever
thorns: treat swellings, ulcers, abscesses in the mouth of children, wounds, skin diseases, indigestion

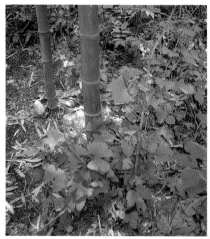

Ginkgo biloba

GLEHNIA
FAMILY: Umbelliferae
Glehnia littoralis 珊瑚菜

The plant is native to Korea, eastern and southeastern China, Taiwan and Japan. In China, the roots are collected, blanched, peeled and dried before use. They taste sweet and have a bitter aftertaste.

Parts used:
roots: improve functioning of the liver and kidneys; treat lung diseases, coughs including hacking cough, fever, chest pain

GLYCYRRHIZA
FAMILY: Leguminosae
Glycyrrhiza glabra 光果甘草
Chinese licorice
licorice
kum cho
sweetwood

This herb is native to the Mediterranean region and central and southwestern Asia. It is grown in southern Europe and southwestern Asia for the roots, which give the licorice of commerce, used in industry as a flavouring and in medicine. This is indicated in its generic name of *Glycyrrhiza* which is Greek for sweet root. The presence of a glycoside, glycyrrhizine, is responsible for the licorice-like taste and for its excessive sweetness, said to be about 50 times sweeter than sugar. Licorice roots are very important in Chinese medicine, second only to ginseng. They are commonly added to many prescriptions to give a pleasant taste. As they are cheap as well as good for a number of ailments, their usage is common. It is believed that prolonged usage can be rejuvenating, although recent studies have shown that it can increase blood pressure.

Licorice is also known to have antitoxic properties. In fact it was used in olden China as an antidote for henbane poisoning. It has also been used as an antidote for datura poisoning. A decoction of licorice with soya bean was also used in 18th century China as an antidote for poisons in general.

More recent research has indeed shown that the roots have a detoxifying effect on cocaine hydrochloride and chloral hydrade, and that it can be used as a remedy for tetanus, diphtheria, snake bites and poisoning by globefish. Recent research on two derivatives of the root has shown that they result in the reduction of the size of peptic ulcers which eventually heal.

Licorice has long been used in Europe as a folk medicine for indigestion and to relieve pain caused by an inflamed stomach. Licorice preparations have been used in cough mixtures and as a

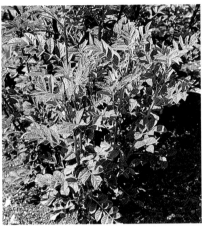
Glycyrrhiza glabra

flavouring for certain medicines. The roots are also used in the confectionery industry and in the curing of tobacco as it imparts a pleasant aroma.

Licorice is not confined to Chinese and European folk medicine. The Africans use an infusion of the stems and roots to treat appendicitis, pulmonary tuberculosis and eye diseases. The Indians use the roots for ailments affecting the bronchial tracts, hoarseness, sore throat and asthma – and for inflammation of the intestinal and urinary tracts. The Vietnamese use the powdered roots as a purgative, a diuretic and to induce sweating.

Parts used:
roots: treat peptic ulcers, general weakness, loss of appetite, cough with the presence of mucus, dizziness, heart palpitation, bleeding haemorrhoids

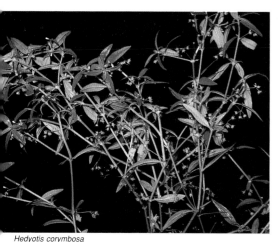
Hedyotis corymbosa

HEDYOTIS
FAMILY: Rubiaceae
Hedyotis
oldenlandia

These are mainly herbs, native to tropical countries. Many are weeds of lawns and waste grounds. About 10 species are used in Chinese medicine.

Hedyotis corymbosa (= Oldenlandia corymbosa) 水线草
two-flowered oldenlandia
This is most commonly used in Chinese medicine. The herbaceous plant has small and narrow leaves, borne sparsely along the slender, profusely branching stem. It has a spreading habit and is commonly found in open places where other weeds do not overgrow it. Flowers are small and white, with usually 2 to 4 blooms at the end of a slender stalk. Although it is believed that this plant can cure cancer, this has not been confirmed by research.

The use of this plant in traditional medicine is seen in cultures other than Chinese. The Malays in Peninsular Malaysia use a poultice of the leaves to treat wounds, sores and sore eyes. The plant is used to control fever in Taiwan, the Philippines and Indochina. In the Philippines the plant is also used as a mouth wash to relieve toothache. In India it is used to treat fever, malaria and nervous depression. In Peninsular Malaysia diffuse oldenlandia (see below) has been reported to have been used as a poultice for lumbago.

Parts used:
leaves, roots: treat inflammation; improve circulation

Hedyotis diffusa 白花蛇舌草
diffuse oldenlandia
Parts used:
juice from plant (excluding roots): treats intestinal diseases
whole plant: treats disorders of the stomach

HIBISCUS
FAMILY: Malvaceae
Hibiscus
hibiscus

Hibiscus is a group of herbs, shrubs and trees from the warm temperate and tropical regions.

The flowers are usually solitary, although sometimes they are in bunches. They are showy and variously coloured – white, yellow, red or purplish.

Hibiscus rosa-sinensis 朱槿
Chinese hibiscus
rose-of-China
Hawaiian hibiscus
China rose
This large shrub originates from Asia, probably China. It is commonly planted in tropical and subtropical countries for the large, showy flowers. Flowers are solitary, usually with red petals but cultivars exist in white, yellow, orange and various shades of red.

Parts used:
leaves, flowers: treat skin diseases, mumps; relieve fever

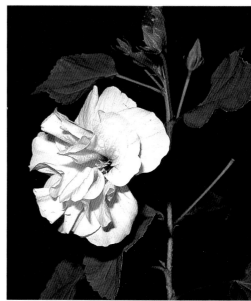
Hibiscus mutabilis

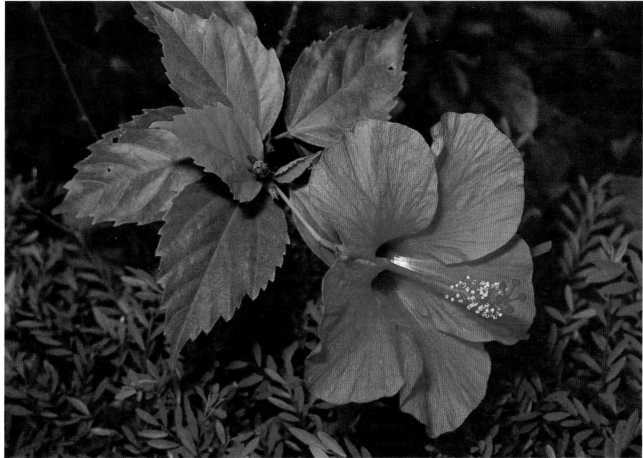

Hibiscus rosa-sinensis

Hibiscus syriacus 木槿
rose-of-sharon

This plant is widely cultivated for its colourful flowers. It is used medicinally for the same purposes in China, Japan and Indochina.

Parts used:
bark, roots, flowers: treat dysentery, indigestion, nausea, internal bleeding

Hibiscus mutabilis 木芙蓉
cotton rose
confederate rose

This hibiscus, from southern China, is often planted as an ornament because of the large and colourful flowers which open white or pink, changing to deep red towards night. The abundant mucilage contained in the tissues makes the plant an effective emollient for burns.

Parts used:
leaves, flowers: pain killer; expel phlegm; treat excessive bleeding during menstruation, painful urination, inflammation, snake bites

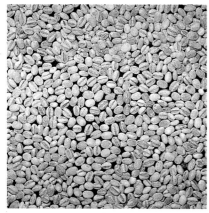

Hordeum vulgare

HORDEUM
FAMILY: Gramineae
Hordeum vulgare 大麦
barley

The generic name comes from the ancient Latin name, *hordeum*, for barley. An annual grass (that is, it lasts only one year), it grows to about 1 m tall. The flowering stalk is erect with conspicuous bristle-like appendages. A native of the temperate Old World, it is now widely cultivated for the grains and as a source of malt. In the tropics barley is planted to a limited extent, especially at high altitudes, for food. Barley is used commercially in the manufacture of beer and whiskey. The dehusked fruits provide the pearl barley of commerce. The seeds, allowed to germinate and then dehydrated, provide us with malt, from which a nourishing drink can be made.

In Chinese medicine the slightly carbonized grains, soaked in boiling water, give a cooling drink.

Parts used:
grains: tonic; aid digestion; induce abortion; expel phlegm

HUMULUS
FAMILY: Cannabaceae
Humulus
hops

Hops are hardy plants, grown as ornaments and for the female flowering heads which give the bitter taste in beer. The hop used in beer production is the common or European hop. The generic name comes from the Latin word, *humus*, "soil", while the specific name for European hop (see below), *lupulus*, means "wolf", because, like the wolf attacking a sheep, the climber embraces the host plant before ultimately strangling it.

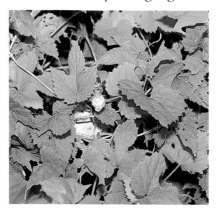

Humulus lupulus

The English name hop is derived from the Anglo-Saxon *hoppan*, "to climb".

Humulus lupulus 啤酒花
European hop
The plant is native to the north temperate regions but has been naturalized elsewhere. It is believed to have been used in beer brewing in the Netherlands in the early 14th century. But its use in England was only seen two centuries later. This was because hops were thought to spoil the flavour of beer as well as endanger the lives of the drinkers. The fruits bear glandular hairs which secrete a chemical known as "bitters", actually lupulin, which imparts the bitter taste in beers. There are male and female plants, but only the latter are cultivated.

Early English herbalists prescribed the seeds as a means of killing intestinal worms. The flowers and fruits were believed to possess the power of expelling poison from the body. Hops stuffed in pillows were believed to induce sleep.

Parts used:
fruits: stimulate gastric activities; increase flow of urine; sedative; bitter tonic

Humulus scandens 葎草
Native of East Asia, this species has greatest usage in Chinese medicine.

Parts used:
leaves: treat coughs, colds
whole plant: treats sores,
premature ejaculation, chronic
dysentery, malaria, typhoid;
increases flow of urine
fruits: treat snake bites,
scorpion stings

HYDNOCARPUS
FAMILY: Flacourtiaceae
Hydnocarpus anthelmintica 大风子
chaulmoogra tree

This is a large tree, native to
Thailand, Burma and India. The
fatty oil extracted from seeds of
most species are used in folk
medicine to treat skin diseases.

Parts used:
seeds: expel intestinal worms;
treat leprosy, elephantiasis,
syphilis, skin diseases
seed oil: treats scabies,
rheumatism, gout

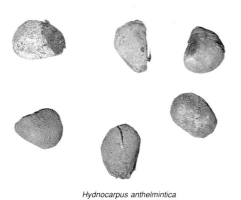

Hydnocarpus anthelmintica

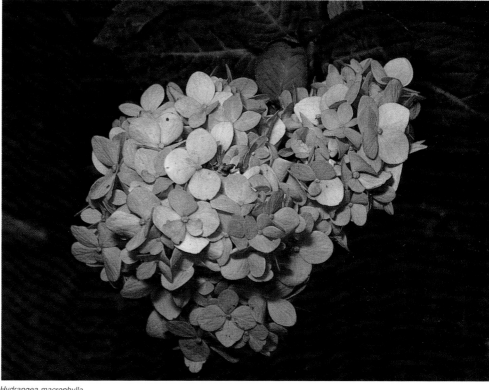

Hydrangea macrophylla

HYDRANGEA
FAMILY: Saxifragaceae
Hydrangea
hydrangea

Hydrangea comes from the the
Greek words *hydros* and *aggos,*
"water" and "jar", or "water
vessel", in reference to the
shape of the fruits. These plants
are deciduous or evergreen
shrubs, native to the Americas
and Asia. Many are garden
ornaments, grown for their
attractive flowers. The American
Indians and later European
settlers, used a decoction of the
plant to remove stones in the
bladder.

Hydrangea aspera spp. *strigosa*
腊莲绣球
Hydrangea heteromalla 八仙花
Parts used:
bark, stem and roots: treat knife
wounds

Hydrangea macrophylla 绣球
Parts used:
flowers: treat malaria; various
heart diseases
leaves, roots: antimalarial drug

95

HYOSCYAMUS
FAMILY: Solanaceae
Hyoscyamus niger 莨菪
henbane
black henbane
stinking nightshade

This is a very poisonous plant, generally grown as an ornament or as a source of the alkaloidal drug hyoscyamine. The generic name, *Hyoscyamus*, is Greek – *hyos*, "hog", *kyamos*, "bean" – for "hog bean", as hogs were said to feed on the fruits. The plant is native to temperate Eurasia. It is covered with sticky hairs and has an odour reminiscent of decaying materials. The flowers are trumpet-shaped and greenish-yellow, with purple veins. The fruit is enclosed within a pitcher-shaped structure, opening by a lid to liberate the many small, brown, kidney-shaped seeds.

Henbane was used by witches in the Middle Ages in Europe to experience hallucination. It was even suggested that the priestesses at the Oracle of Delphi made their prophetic declarations under the influence of smoke from henbane seeds. When burned the fumes were believed to conjure up spirits of the dead and give one the power of clairvoyance.

All parts of the plant are poisonous, especially the leaves and seeds. Poisoning results in drying of the mouth, impaired speech, dilated pupils and blindness. These symptoms are soon followed by excitement, stupor with low blood pressure, difficulty in breathing, unconsciousness and, finally, death. The symptoms may include double vision, fits of rage and aggressiveness. This plant has in fact been used since ancient times as a poison and a pain killer.

European herbalists used to boil the leaves in wine and used the solution to reduce swellings in the scrotum and breasts, and to soothe gout and aching joints. Leaves were soaked in vinegar and then applied to the forehead, to relieve headache. Bathing one's feet in a bath of the plant before going to bed was believed to cure insomnia.

Parts used:
seeds: pain killer; narcotic; treat muscular pain, coughs, asthma, epilepsy, toothache, spasms

ILLICIUM
Illicium verum 八角茴香
star anise
true anise

This is so named because of the star-shaped fruit. The generic name, *Illicium*, is Latin, meaning "allurement" or "that which entices", in reference to the agreeable scent of the plant. The plant is a slow-growing tree, native to the mountains of southern China and northeastern Vietnam. Leaves are aromatic and flowers whitish, turning pink, then purple. The star-shaped fruits ripen red, splitting along each segment to expose the glossy, brown seed. The plant is grown for its aromatic fruits which are collected unripe and used as a culinary spice to flavour curries, confectionery and other foods. It is also used to aromatize cordials and liqueurs like anisette. An oil, distilled from the fruits, is used in medicine and for flavouring.

Parts used:
fruit oil: antidote for a number of poisons; treats rheumatism

Illicium anisatum 八角茴香
Chinese anise
Japanese anise
This evergreen tree, native to Japan and southern Korea, has been known to be poisonous since early times and has been used as a fish and rat poison. It is not used internally.

Parts used:
plant: treats skin problems

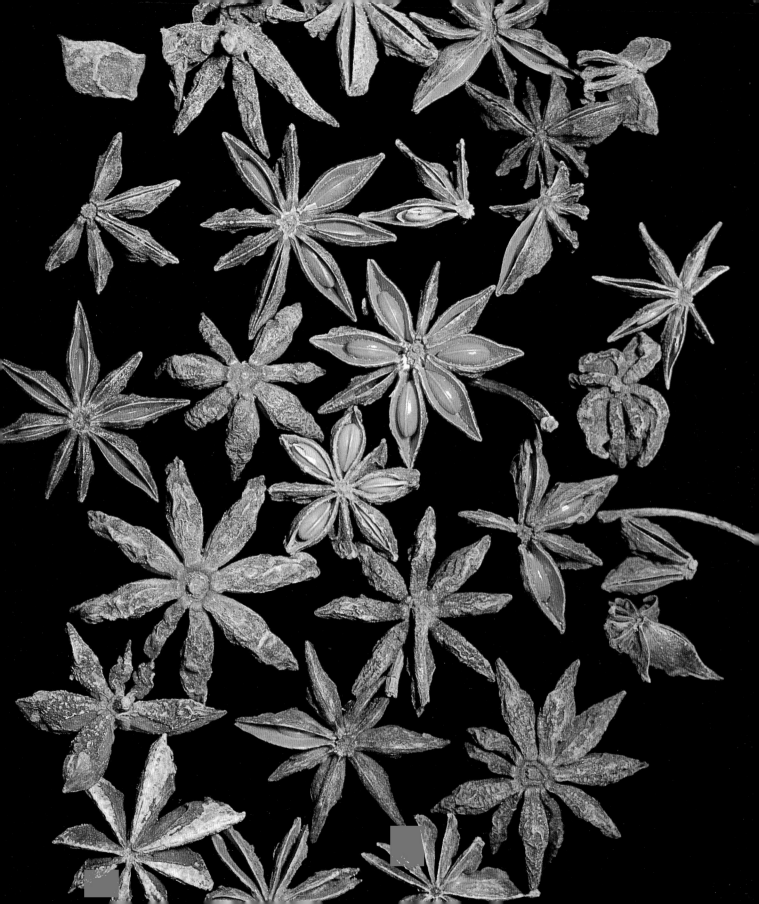

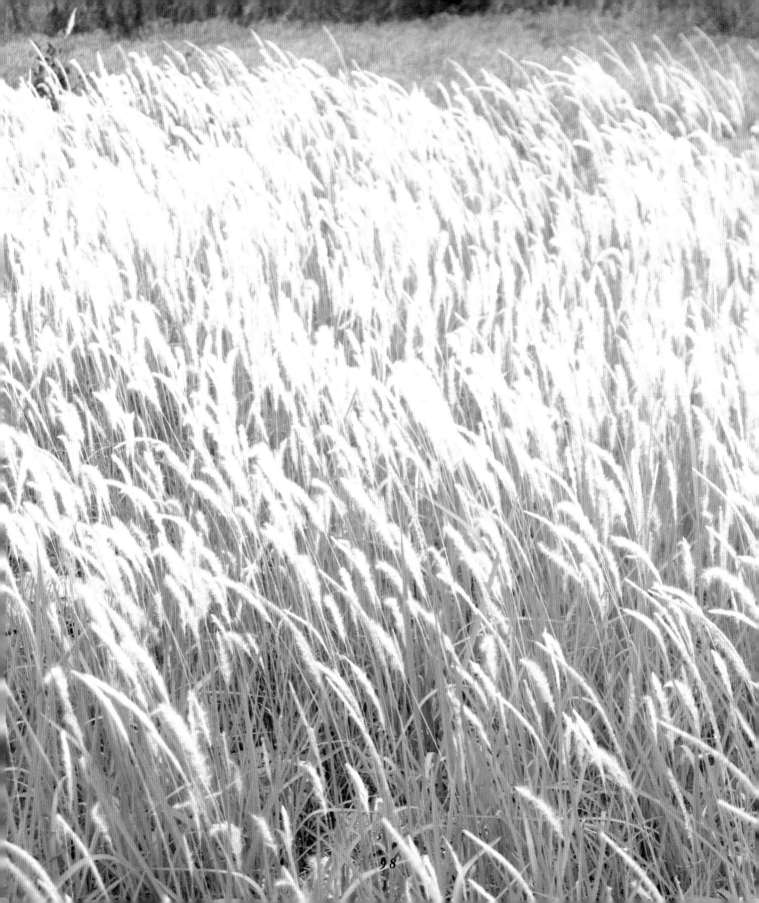

Imperata cylindrica

IMPERATA
FAMILY: Gramineae
Imperata cylindrica 白茅根
lalang

The generic name of lalang, *Imperata*, honours Ferrante Imperato of Naples, a physician and naturalist. Lalang is a weedy grass of pantropic distribution, covering disturbed areas where the soil has been degraded through bad cultural practices. The sharp, erect blades of the leaves, totally covering the ground, are easily burnt. Regular fires during dry periods burn off the leaves but the underground stems survive, sprouting new leaves and flowering shoots. The fire helps to maintain the purity of the grass cover, killing off any other plants that have managed to grow among these plants. Firing also stimulates flowering and this no doubt helps to disperse the plant far and wide.

The slender stems, roots and flowers are all used in Chinese medicine. Various parts of the plant have also been used as herbal remedies in Japan, Indochina, Peninsular Malaysia, Indonesia and the Philippines. Extracts of the plant have been shown to have antiviral property. They have also been reported to have anticancer properties when tested on animals.

Parts used:
roots: stop bleeding; treat fever, acute inflammation of the kidneys, cough with phlegm
underground stem: treats influenza, blood in the urine, internal bleeding, jaundice, coughs, kidney diseases, coughing of blood
flowers: treat blood in the sputum, nose bleeds, lung diseases; quench thirst

INDIGOFERA
FAMILY: Leguminosae
Indigofera tinctoria 木蓝
indigo

The generic name of indigo is Latin for "indigo bearing", as the plant yields a blue dye, the indigo of commerce. The plant is a widely distributed shrub, native to the tropics.

Parts used:
plant: treats diseases of the liver, dysentery

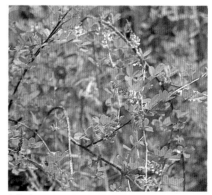

Indigofera

99

INULA
FAMILY: Compositae
Inula

Inula are herbs, native to the temperate and subtropical regions in the Old World. The stem is often covered with hairs which may be glandular.

Inula britannica 旋复花
This plant is native to northern China, Manchuria, Mongolia and Korea.

Parts used:
plant, roots: relieve attacks of bronchitis, hay fever and asthma

Inula helenium 土木香
elecampane
The plant is native to central Asia.

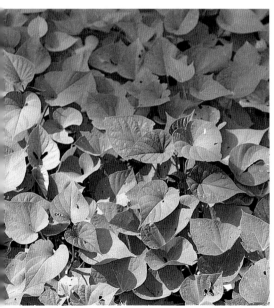

Ipomoea batatas

Parts used:
roots: expel intestinal worms; treat cholera, malarial fever, dysentery, bronchitis, snake bites, insect stings

IPOMOEA
FAMILY: Convolvulaceae
Ipomoea
ipomoea

Ipomoeas are twining, prostrate plants, native to tropical and warm temperate regions. Many are ornamental and some have hallucinogenic properties. The sweet potato is the most important member, yielding the edible root crop.

Ipomoea batatas 番薯
sweet potato
This is a tropical American plant, brought to Europe by Columbus. The Spanish and the Portuguese in turn brought the plant to the East. It is now widely grown in many tropical and subtropical countries for their tuberous roots, which are used as food. In fact it is an important food crop in many countries, where the leaves may also be eaten as a vegetable. The roots are also used as stock feed or for industrial purposes.

Parts used:
roots: tonic for the stomach, spleen and kidneys

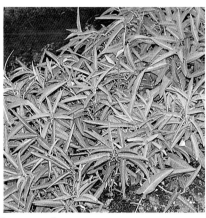

Ipomoea aquatica

Ipomoea aquatica 蕹菜
kangkong
This is grown as a vegetable but is also used medicinally by the Chinese. Cooked with pork, the plant is prescribed for general weakness, yellowish discharge from the vagina and cough.

Parts used:
plant: tonic; laxative; antidote for certain food poisoning

Ipomoea hederacea 牵牛子
Native to tropical America, the plant is now a weed of wastelands and waysides in many tropical and subtropical countries. The dried mature seeds, which taste bitter, are reported to be poisonous and to have hallucinogenic properties. In a number of Asian countries the plant is used mainly as a purgative while the seeds are used for constipation and to induce menstruation and

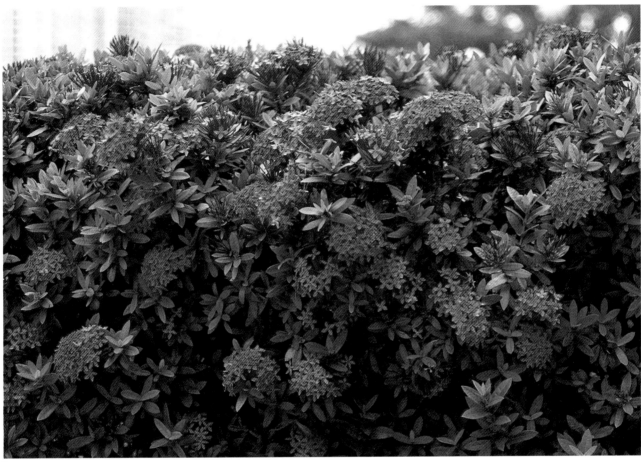

Ixora

abortion. The use of the plant as a purgative has scientific support in that many *Ipomoea* species have been known to contain compounds in their underground roots which have purgative properties.

Parts used:
seeds: treat constipation; increase flow of urine; expel intestinal worms

IXORA
FAMILY: Rubiaceae
Ixora chinensis 龙船花
Chinese ixora

The name ixora comes from a Malabar deity. These are evergreen shrubs or small trees of the tropics. There are many attractive wild species that have yet to be brought into cultivation. Those that are in

cultivation are handsome plants, as their flowers are brightly coloured and their foliage attractive. This plant is native to southern China and Peninsular Malaysia, bearing dense clusters of yellow flowers which turn orange-red with age.

Parts used:
whole plant: treats rheumatism, abscesses, bruises; relieves pain

101

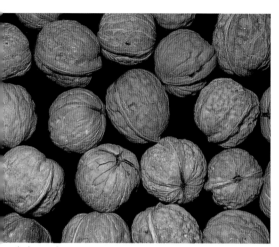

Juglans regia

JUGLANS
FAMILY: Juglandaceae
Juglans regia 胡桃
walnut
English walnut
Persian walnut

The generic name, *Juglans*, is derived from the ancient Latin name *Jovis glans* or the "nut of Jupiter". To the Greeks and Romans of antiquity, the walnut was a symbol of fertility, and was served at weddings and feasts. According to the doctrine of signatures, the convoluted shell of the walnut made it suitable for the treatment of brain disorders. European herbalists used the juice of the unripe fruits, mixed with honey, as a gargle for sore throat; the bark as a purgative; the husk and shell of the nut to cause sweating; and the oil extracted from the ripe kernels for colic, wounds and skin diseases.

Native to western Asia and southeastern Europe, the tree is found throughout Europe and Asia. It is also grown for the edible fruit and the fine-grained wood, much used for furniture, and as ornaments. Walnut oil is used by painters as a drying oil. The green husk of the fruit gives a yellow dye while the leaves a brown one, the latter sometimes used as a hair dye.

Parts used:
kernel: tonic; increase flow of urine
kernel oil: mild purgative; treats skin diseases; expels intestinal worms
leaves: treat conjunctivitis

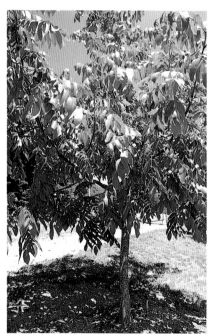

Juglans regia

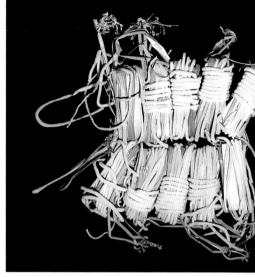

Juncus effusus

JUNCUS
FAMILY: Juncaceae
Juncus effusus var. *decipiens* 灯心草
bog rush
Japanese-mat rush

The plant grows up to 1 m high, in a dense mass. The short-creeping rootstock bears few brownish, scale-like leaves, which are found towards the base of the stem. Flowers are solitary, small and light green. The plants grow in wet locations in the lowlands and mountains of Japan, China, Korea and North America. In Japan it is cultivated for use in the weaving of tatami, the standard floor covering of Japanese homes. In China the stem pith is used as wicks for lamps and for the making of mats.

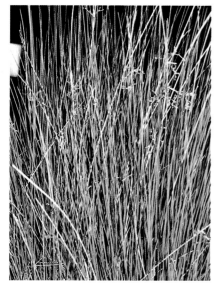

Juncus effusus

Parts used:
pith: purgative; sedative; treats insomnia, inflammation of the throat, coughs, loss of memory

JUNIPERUS
FAMILY: Cupressaceae
Juniperus chinensis 圓柏
Chinese juniper

Chinese juniper is an evergreen conifer of temperate East Asia. The leaves are tiny and set very closely on the twigs. The juvenile leaves are needlelike and spiny, while the adult leaves are scale-like.

Parts used:
leaves: tonic to treat bleeding resulting from coughs

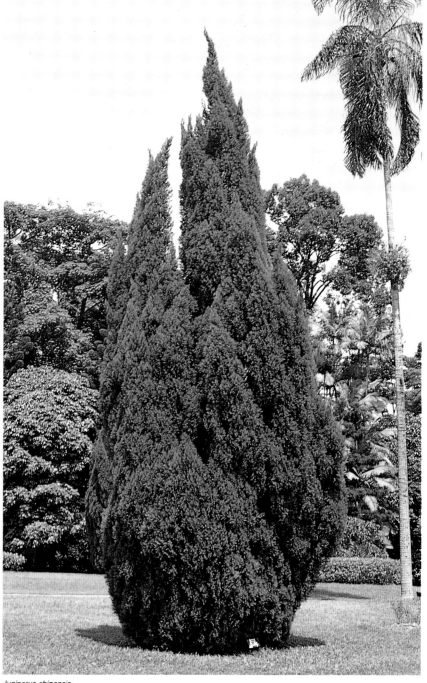

Juniperus chinensis

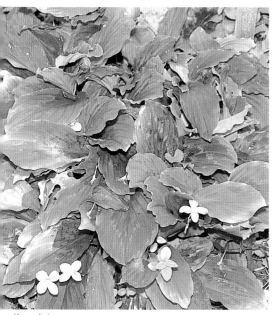

Kaempferia

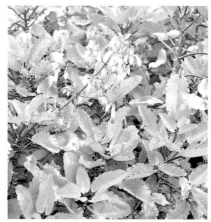

Kalanchoe pinnata

KNOXIA
FAMILY: Rubiaceae

Knoxia corymbosa
knoxia

The slender, erect herb, native to India, is named after R. Knox, a traveller and resident of Sri Lanka. Its small, white or purple flowers are clustered at the end of the stalk, while the leaves are long and rough.

Parts used:
tuberous roots: treat ailments of the excretory system, inflammation, dropsy of the abdomen

LANTANA
Family: Verbenaceae

Lantana camara 马缨丹
lantana
yellow sage

To the Malays the plant is known as *bunga tahi ayam* as the leaves tend to remind them of chicken droppings. A native of tropical America, this shrub is now naturalized in many countries, often occurring as a weed. The flowers are in flat-topped heads, appearing orange-yellow or orange and changing in colour to red or white.

Parts used:
whole plant: bath for scabies and leprosy

KAEMPFERIA
FAMILY: Zingiberaceae

Kaempferia galanga 山奈
kaempferia

This is a herb of the Old World tropics, cultivated in many Southeast Asian countries. The plant has been used for flavouring rice and the roots to make cosmetics.

Parts used:
underground stems: stimulant; treat toothache, cholera, chest pains, headache, constipation

KALANCHOE
FAMILY: Crassulacese

Kalanchoe pinnata 落地生根
life plant
leaf plant
air plant
Mexican love plant
sprouting leaf
good luck leaf

The many common names of this plant reflect on the ability of the leaves to produce young plants once detached from the parent plant. The leaves are favourites with children who love to place them between the pages of a book until the young shoots sprout and give roots. The plant is pantropic in distribution.

Parts used:
leaves: treat boils, wounds, burns, scalds, skin diseases, headache, coughs

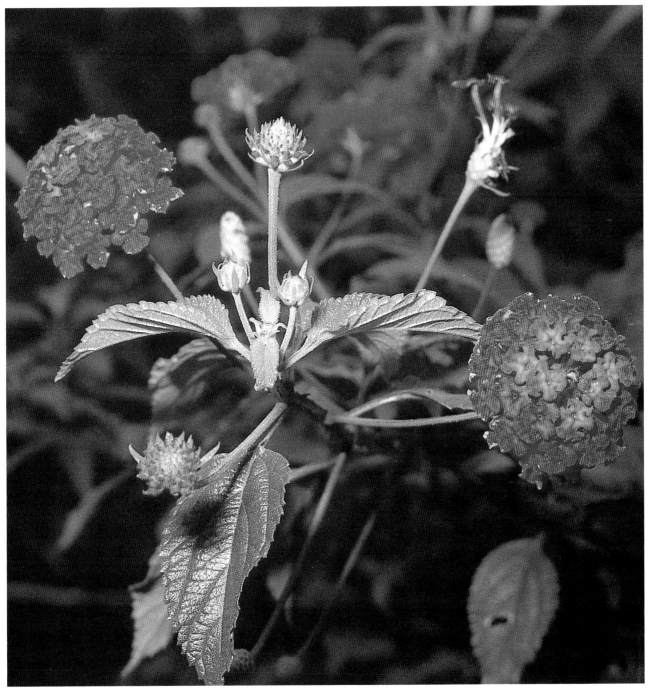

Lantana camara

LEONURUS
Family: Labiatae
Leonurus sibiricus 益母草
motherwort

Motherwort is *Leonurus*, from the Greek *leon* for "lion" and *ouros* for "tail", as the plant was thought to resemble the tail of a lion. European herbalists consider the plant the herb of life and prescribe it for the treatment of chest complaints, urinary disorders, cramps and convulsions. The Chinese make use of the sweet and pungent seeds for various ailments. This herb is native to northeastern Asia, Japan and Taiwan.

Parts used:
seeds: aid in urination; cool the body system; treat excessive menstrual flow, absence of menstruation

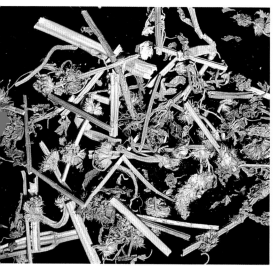

Leonurus

LEPIDIUM
FAMILY: Cruciferae
Lepidium apetalum 独行菜
peppergrass

A herb of the temperate regions, the plant is rich in mucilage, which could be responsible for its effectiveness in the treatment of coughs. Certain species have shown antibacterial properties.

Parts used:
roots: treat common cold, cough, choking of the chest, excess sputum

LIGUSTICUM
FAMILY: Umbelliferae
Ligusticum striatum
lovage

According to the legends and folklore of several countries, lovage is reputed to be one of the ingredients in love potions.

Parts used:
roots: treat gout, rheumatism; relieve pain; increase menstrual flow; sedative for headache; improve blood circulation

LIGUSTRUM
FAMILY: Oleaceae
Ligustrum lucidum 女贞
glossy privet
Nepal privet
white wax tree

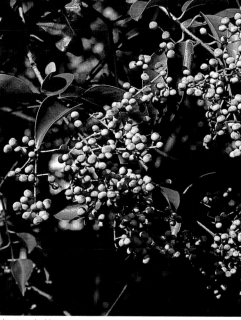

Ligustrum lucidum

This is an evergreen tree, native to China, Korea and Japan. The tree is commonly planted along roads for their attractive foliage and profusion of small, white flowers. The generic name, *Ligustrum*, is Latin for "privet". However, there are others who believe that the name comes from the Latin word *ligo*, "I bind", in reference to the use of the twigs to make baskets.

Parts used:
bark: promotes sweating
leaves: promote sweating; treat coughs, swellings, dizziness, headache, fever; pain killer
fruits: tonic; prolong life

106

LILIUM
FAMILY: Liliaceae
Lilium brownii var. *colchesteri* 百合
lily

This plant is from central China. It is bulbous and bears slightly fragrant flowers which are pure white on the inside and rose-purple on the outside. The scales of the bulbs are blanched and dried and then bleached with sulphur fumes before use.

Parts used:
bulb scales: sedative; tonic; treat cough, lung disorders, urinary disorders, deafness, earache, nervousness, excessive gas in the system

LINDERA
FAMILY: Lauraceae
Lindera strychnifolia 乌药
lindera

The generic name, *Lindera*, commemorates the Swedish physician J. Linder (1676–1723). The plant is an aromatic shrub from central China and Taiwan.

Parts used:
roots: tonic for urinary system; expel intestinal worms; treat inflammation of the abdomen and chest, hernia, indigestion, asthma, stomach spasms, cholera, painful menstruation

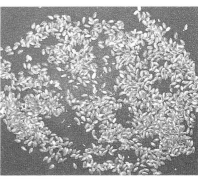
Linum usitatissimum

LINUM
FAMILY: Linaceae
Linum usitatissimum 亚麻
flax

Linum is Latin for flax. The plant is one of the oldest under cultivation and references to it are found in the Old as well as the New Testament. The "fine linen" mentioned in the Bible has been satisfactorily proved to have been spun flax. Flax is a graceful little plant with turquoise-blue flowers, native probably to Asia. It is widely grown in temperate countries for its fibres, derived from the stem, from which flax fibre and fine linen are obtained. The plant is also cultivated for the seeds, from which linseed oil and linseed cake and meal are manufactured.

European herbalists used the seeds to make a tea prescribed as a cure for coughs and bronchial problems, and inflammation of the urinary organs, lungs and bowels. The plant itself was used to treat piles and dysentery.

Parts used:
linseed meal: poultice
oil: emollient; purgative

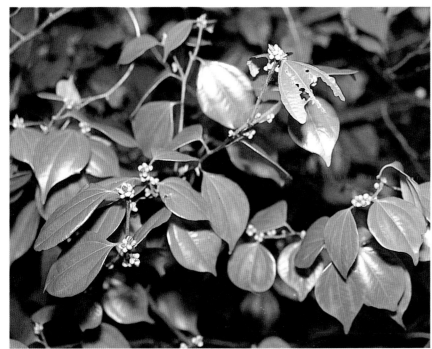
Lindera strychnifolia

Liquidambar formosana

LIQUIDAMBAR
FAMILY: Hamamelidaceae
Liquidambar formosana 枫香树
Formosan gum
Formosan sweet gum

The generic name, *Liquidambar* is derived from the Latin *liquidus* for "fluid" and Arabic *ambar* for "amber", in reference to the fragrant resin obtained from the bark. The tree is tall and deciduous, native to southern China and Taiwan and planted in Japan. Leaves are simple but three-lobed, the lobing radiating from the point of attachment to the slender stalk. Flowers are reduced, the male growing on separate trees from the female. Fruits are round, spiny heads, splitting open at maturity to liberate the winged seeds. The resin is collected from old trees and dried in the sun until it becomes yellow, transparent and brittle. It is bitter and pungent and, when burnt, very aromatic.

Parts used:
resin: aids blood circulation; suppresses bleeding; stops pain; helps wounds to heal; inhibits bleeding; treats boils, headache
fruits: treat lumbago, skin diseases, articular pains
bark: treats skin diseases
roots, leaves: treat cancerous growths

LIRIOPE
FAMILY: Liliaceae
Liriope spicata 大叶麦冬
creeping lily-turf

The genus is named after the nymph Liriope. The herb is native to China and Japan. It possesses slender, jointed rootstocks, from which arise stiff, grasslike leaves, in clumps. Flowers are violet-blue and showy, and borne on a simple stalk growing from the centre of the bunch of leaves, the stalk generally longer than the leaves. These develop into blue berries, each with a few black seeds.

Parts used:
underground stems: expel phlegm from respiratory passages; treat coughs

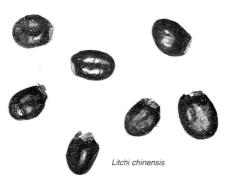
Litchi chinensis

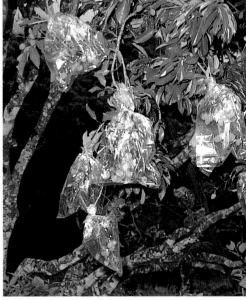
Litchi chinensis

LITCHI
FAMILY: Sapindaceae
Litchi chinensis 荔枝
lychee
litchi

This is a well known fruit which originates from southern China. It is now widely grown in the tropics and subtropics for its fresh as well as dried fruits. The fruits are roundish, bright red when ripe, and have a white and fleshy edible layer over the black seed.

Parts used:
fresh fruits: tonic, treat cough, diarrhoea
fruits together with skin and leaves: treat bites from poisonous animals
seeds: pain killer; tonic; thirst quencher; treat hernia, lumbago, ulcers, inflammation of the testicles

LITHOSPERMUM
FAMILY: Boraginaceae
Lithospermum erythrorhizon 紫草
gromwell

Gromwell is often planted for the roots, which give a purple dye. The generic name, *Lithospermum* comes from the Greek words *lithos*, "stone", and *sperma*, "seed", as the seeds of these plants are like small stones. This highly hairy herb is from northern China and Japan.

Parts used:
roots: purgative; treat cuts and burns, fever, stomach disorders including constipation, skin eruptions, insect stings, smallpox; increase flow of urine

LOBELIA
FAMILY: Campanulaceae
Lobelia chinensis 半边莲
lobelia

Lobelia is named after Matthias de Lobel, a Flemish botanist and author (1538–1616). Native mainly to tropical and warm temperate countries, it is grown in borders of flower beds. Most lobelias have lobeline and related alkaloids. Pure lobeline is used in modern medicine to treat respiratory problems in newly born babies, during anaesthesia and to relieve asthmatic symptoms. The chemical is also used in preparations for smokers wanting to kick the habit. It is poisonous and, in high dosage, can have paralytic effect, resulting in vomiting and collapse.

Parts used:
whole plant: treats snake bite poisoning, wasp and scorpion stings, boils

LONICERA
FAMILY: Caprifoliaceae
Lonicera japonica 忍冬
Japanese honeysuckle
gold-and-silver flower
honeysuckle

Lonicera is named in honour of Adam Lonicer, a German physician and naturalist (1528–1586). The common name, honeysuckle, was given in the mistaken belief that bees obtained honey from the flowers. In ancient Greece the plant was an object of religious

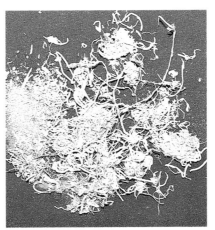
Lobelia chinensis

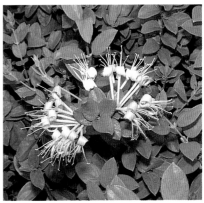
Lonicera japonica

worship. European herbalists used to squeeze the juice from the plant to treat snake bites. The seeds and flowers, boiled and mixed with oil, are applied to swellings. The flowers are still being used as a cure for asthma. The leaves have been reported to be poisonous but this claim is controversial. Pharmacological studies have shown the plant to have the capability of increasing as well as reducing blood sugar content and to have antitumour, antibacterial and antifungal properties.

The plant has white or purplish fragrant flowers, occurring in pairs. A number of cultivars exist, each with differently coloured leaves. Native to East Asia, the plant has become naturalized in North America.

Parts used:
whole plant: increases flow of urine; reduces fever; prevents diarrhoea
flowers: treat fever, headache, diarrhoea, inflammation, arthritis, dysentery
twigs: treat aching bones, boils

LOPHATHERUM
FAMILY: Gramineae

Lophatherum gracile 淡竹叶
crested grass

The generic name is derived from the Greek words *lophos*, "crest" or "tuft", and *thrix*, "hair" or "bristle", in reference to the tuft of bristle on the sterile bracts. This grass is about 1 m high and commonly found along paths in lowland and hill forests. The plant is tufted, bearing sparingly branched flowering heads, the branches in turn bearing a number of closely spaced secondary heads. The inconspicuous florets develop into fruitlets, each with a number of bristle-like structures which stick to clothings of people or to animals, who thus assist in their dispersal. The grass is widely distributed throughout Asia and Australia.

Parts used:
whole plant: treats fever, anxiety, abnormally small amount of urine, blood in the urine; cools the body system; purgative
roots: induce abortion; aid and hasten difficult labour

LORANTHUS
FAMILY: Loranthaceae

Loranthus
mistletoe

Loranthus are green, semi-parasitic shrubs that grow on the branches of trees, tapping nutrients from the host. The leaves of these plants are simple and leathery or sometimes reduced to scales. The flowers are mostly small, and yellow or red, developing into small berries with sticky pulp. These berries are sought after by birds, which help in their distribution.

According to an ancient legend, the cross on which Christ was crucified was made from the wood of mistletoe. As punishment, the plant was banished from this earth and thus had to depend on the goodwill of other plants to survive. In Brittany the plant is called Herbe de la Croix. Mistletoe, together with holly and ivy, are associated with Christmas in England and certain European countries. The tradition of kissing under the Christmas mistletoe could probably be associated with powers of the plant to increase fertility. It was during the pre-Christian era when the Druids, the ancient order of priests in Gaul, Britain and Ireland, became aware of the fruitfulness of the plant in midwinter. Subsequently, European herbalists prescribed the plant to childless couples to assist in conception, to the unmarried to increase their chances of marriage, and as a cure for

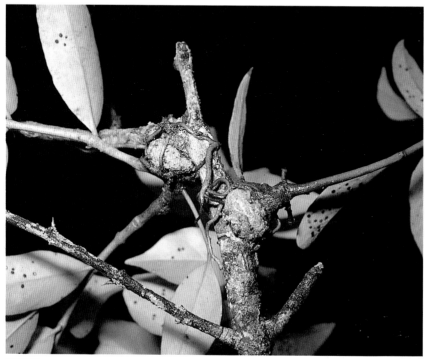

Loranthus

sterility. The plant has also been used to cure epilepsy and other convulsive nervous disorders, to check internal bleeding and to treat urinary disorders, rheumatism, gout and heart disease.

Modern taxonomists have split *Loranthus* into a number of genera, but for convenience, their old scientific names are given, with the new names between parentheses.

Loranthus parasiticus (Scurrula parasitica) 桑寄生
Parts used:
whole plant: tonic for kidneys; induces secretion of milk in women after birth; strengthens the bones; relieves pain in the back and knees; reduces high blood pressure; relieves soreness of the limbs and lumbar, pains of pregnant women

Loranthus yadoriki (Taxillus yadoriki) 毛叶桑寄生
Parts used:
twigs, leaves: induce secretion of milk in women after birth; quieten the pregnant uterus; treat excessive menstrual bleeding, threatened abortion; pain killer

LUFFA
FAMILY: Cucurbitaceae
Luffa aegyptiaca 丝瓜
sponge gourd
dishcloth gourd
smooth loofah
si gua

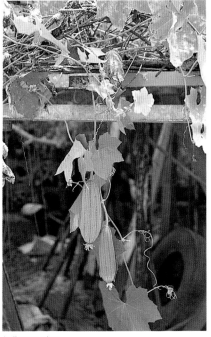
Luffa aegyptiaca

The sponge gourd is so called because the fibrous fruit is used as a sponge. It is an annual (that is, it lasts only one year) herbaceous vine of the Old World tropics, widely cultivated for the fruit, either to be eaten or used. Branched tendrils assist the slender stem to scramble upwards. The sponge gourd fruits are nearly cylindrical, with small, flat, black seeds, bordered by a narrow wing. These seeds yield an edible oil. The interior of the fruit is used as a bath sponge or a general cleaning sponge. It has also been made into table mats, bath mats, sandals and gloves. In the United States, before the last world war, it was used in engine filters. Because of its shock and sound absorbing properties, it was used in steel helmets and armoured vehicles in the United States army. The sap from the stem is used in toilet preparations in Japan and in native medicines in the East. The fruit juice is a powerful purgative; it is toxic.

Parts used:
fibre of fruit: pain killer; stops bleeding in the treatment of dysentery; treats excessive bleeding from the uterus, piles, inflammation of the testicles
ash from the fibres: cooling drink; aids blood circulation; increases menstrual flow; arrests internal bleeding; treats smallpox, jaundice, cancerous swellings, hiccups

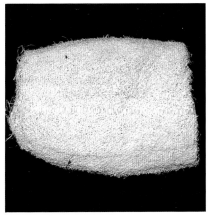
Luffa aegyptiaca

111

LYCIUM
FAMILY: Solanaceae
Lycium
matrimony vine
box thorn

Matrimony vines are shrubs, native to the tropics or warm temperate regions, often growing in dry areas.

Lycium barbarum 宁夏枸杞
The plant is a spreading or upright herb, with spiny branches. It is native to the region stretching from North Africa to Iraq.

Parts used:
fruits, root bark: treat impotence, backache, dizziness, general weakness, fever

Lycium chinense 枸杞
Chinese wolfberry
Chinese matrimony vine
This is native to China and Japan but now naturalized in Europe and the United States.

Parts used:
fruits: treat impotence, backache, dizziness, general weakness, fever, diabetes
root bark: treats impotence, backache, dizziness, general weakness, fever, sore throat, rheumatism, fever, pneumonia

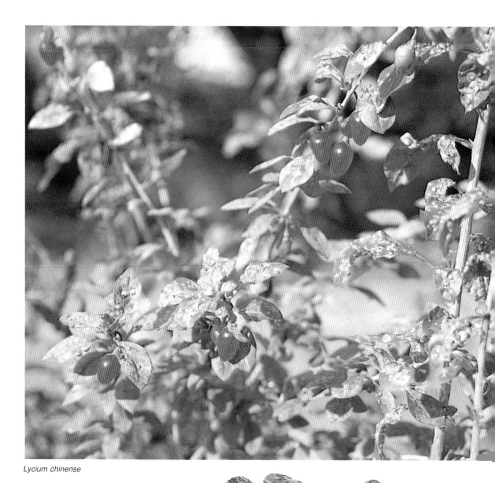

Lycium chinense

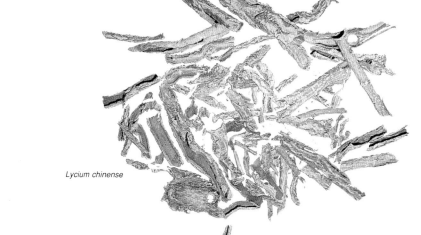

Lycium chinense

LYCOPODIUM
FAMILY: Lycopodiaceae
Lycopodium cernuum 垂穗万松
nodding clubmoss
rumput serani
paku serani

The generic name is derived from the Greek words – *lykos*, "wolf", and *podion*, "foot" – for wolf-foot, because of its resemblance to a wolf's foot. The plant is found growing in open grounds under the full sun, especially where the soil is poor. The stem is thin and scrambling, covered with spirally-arranged scale-like leaves. At the tips of certain branches are the cones, bearing spore sacs. Because the spores have a high oil content and they burn easily, they were used in the production of artificial lighting in olden theatres, in photographic flash and in gunpowder. In fireworks the spores provide the bright blaze and the continuous crackling sound. In olden days the spores were used to dust over pills so as to keep them from sticking together and to disguise their flavour. Locally, the plant is used in the making of wreaths and in flower arrangement.

Parts used:
plant: treats burns, dysentery, hepatitis, rheumatism, sore eyes, traumatic injuries

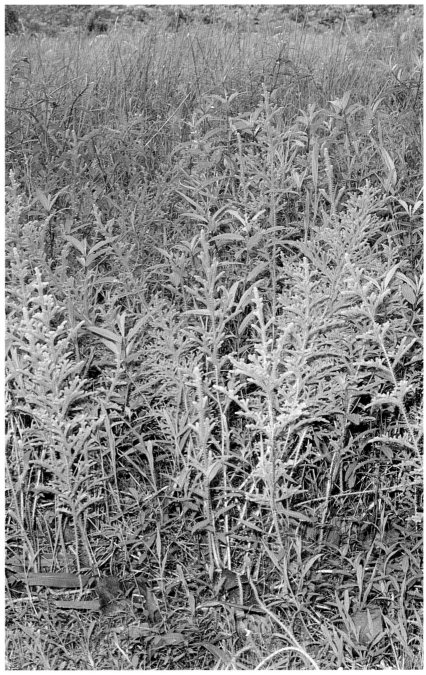

Lycopodium cernuum

LYGODIUM
FAMILY: Schizaeaceae
Lygodium
climbing fern

The generic name, *Lygodium*, is Greek for flexible, no doubt referring to the twining leaves of the plant. The fern has an underground stem, which bears, at regular intervals, the twining leaves. These leaves consist of a thin and elongated twining structure from which arises the leaflets. Fertile leaflets bear narrow lobes which in turn bear spore sacs. The twining leaves are twisted into crude ropes, used in villages or used to plait baskets or as a weaving material for handbags.

Lygodium japonicum
Japanese climbing fern 海金沙
Parts used:
leaves: treat coughing with blood, gonorrhoea; sedative in the treatment of high fever and delirium

Lygodium flexuosum 曲轴海金沙
Parts used:
leaves: internal medicine to clear inflammation; relieve inflammation of the bladder; hasten the maturity of smallpox pustules
spores: treat fever

Lygodium flexuosum

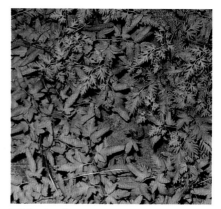

Lygodium japonicum

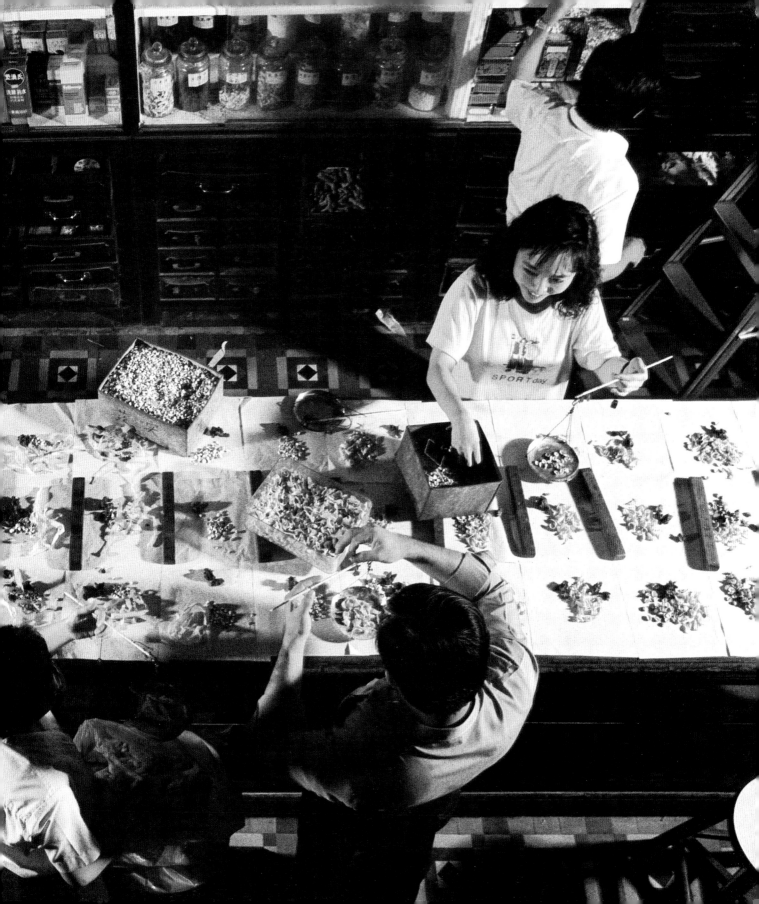

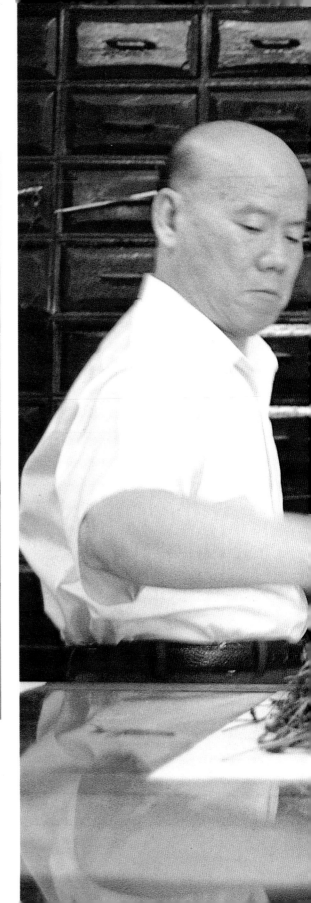

The expert hand of the master herbalist quickly gathers the right measure of herbs for a decoction.

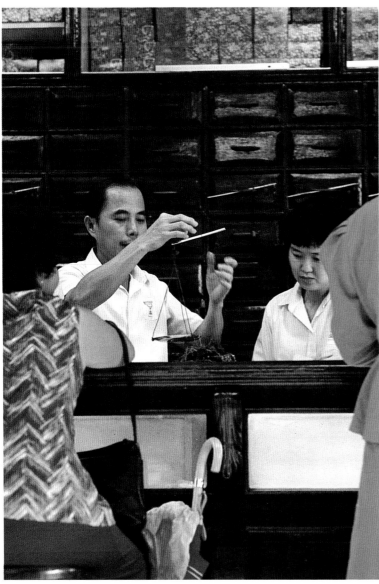

Behind the highly polished counter, herbalists gather, weigh and combine prescriptions for customers.

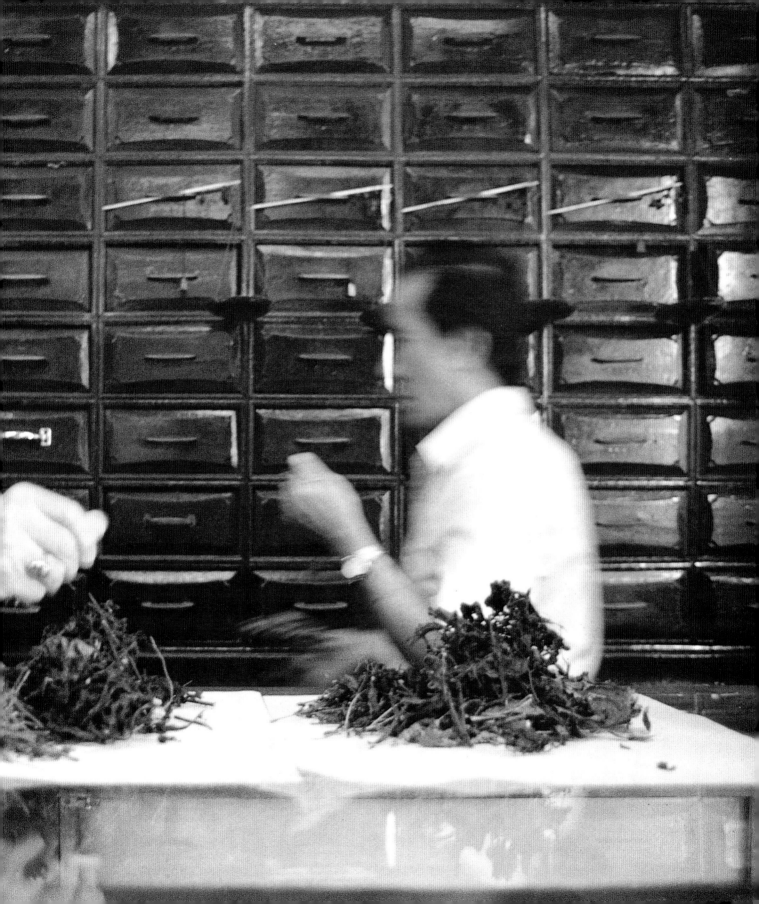

MAGNOLIA
FAMILY: Magnoliaceae
Magnolia
magnolia

These are deciduous and evergreen trees and shrubs, native to Asia and the Americas. The leaves are often leathery while the flowers are large, solitary and showy – white, pink, purple or yellow. Many such trees are planted as ornaments in gardens and to line roads. Magnolia is named after Pierre Magnol (1638–1715), a botanist from Montpelier, France.

Magnolia officinalis 厚朴
This is a deciduous tree, native to western China but extensively cultivated. The flowers are large, white and fragrant. The fragrant bark is collected for its medicinal value. Stripped of its bark, the tree usually dies.

Parts used:
bark: antispasmodic; aphrodisiac; expels phlegm from respiratory passages; expels intestinal worms; treats spastic gastritis, peptic ulcer, diarrhoea, vomiting, typhoid fever, malaria, loss of appetite, shortness of breath, coughs, nausea
flower buds: increase menstrual flow

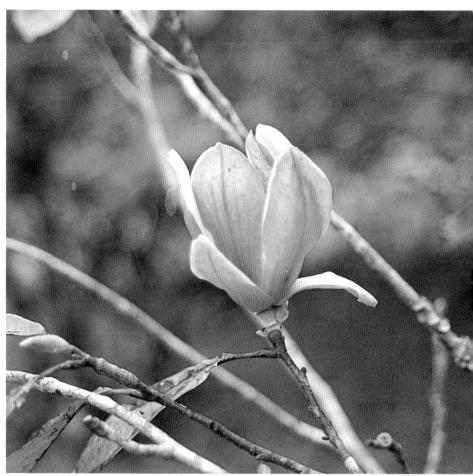

Magnolia

Magnolia quinquepeta 辛夷
This is a native Chinese magnolia, a deciduous shrub with large, bell-shaped, fragrant flowers whose petals are purple on the outside and white on the inside.

Parts used:
flower buds: tonic; pain killer

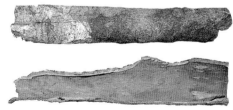

Magnolia

MELIA
FAMILY: Meliaceae

Melia azedarach 苦楝
chinaberry
chinaberry tree
China tree
pride-of-India
pride-of-China
Persian lilac
Indian lilac
bead tree
paradise tree

This is an attractive wayside tree with fern-like foliage, native to Asia. The fruits are poisonous and six to eight seeds can kill a man. There have been isolated reports from many parts of the world of people being poisoned as a result of eating the fruit. Domestic animals such as pigs, sheep and goats have also been poisoned by the fruit. Besides the fruits, the leaves, flowers and bark have also been reported to be poisonous. The plant has been used as a fish poison as well as an insecticide. Leaves placed between the covers of books help to keep insects away. The bony seeds are threaded by monks and others to make rosaries, hence the common name, bead tree.

Parts used:
fruits, stem, bark: purgative; treat chest and abdominal pains; expel intestinal worms; induce vomiting

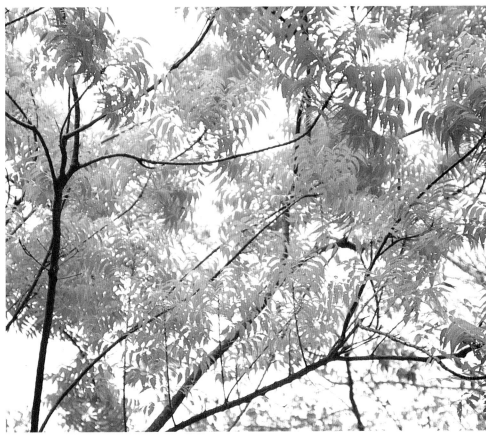
Melia azedarach

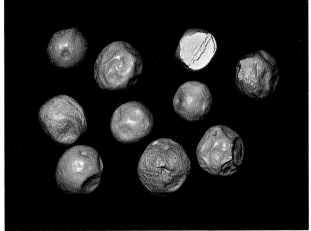
Melia azedarach

MENTHA
FAMILY: Labiatae
Mentha
mints

The generic name comes from the Greek name of a nymph, Minte. Mints, of which there are many, are usually cultivated for their aromatic essential oils contained in all parts of the plant. The field mint, a native of the northern hemisphere, is a hairy perennial herb, easily recognized from its aromatic leaves. Flowers are small and lilac, white or sometimes pink. The Japanese mint, which is a variety of this species, is an important source of menthol.

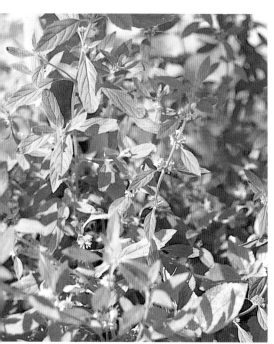

Mentha arvensis

Mentha arvensis 薄荷
field mint
Parts used:
whole plant: pain killer; removes excessive gas in the system; induces sweating; stimulates gastric activities; treats sore throat, common cold, headache, inflammation of the eyes and of the skin, cold sores, toothache, cancer, cardiovascular disorders

Mentha x piperita 留兰香
peppermint
This grows everywhere in China.

Parts used:
leaves: treat upset stomach, nausea, vomiting; remove excessive gas from the system

METROXYLON
FAMILY: Palmae
Metroxylon sagu 西谷椰子
sago palm

Sago palm is native to the Moluccas and West New Guinea. It is now widely cultivated in freshwater swamps for the sago and the leaves, used for thatching. The palm develops in clumps, with suckers, or young palms, growing from the base of the main palm. Usually, after 15 years, the palm produces a huge terminal flowering branch, after which it dies and slowly

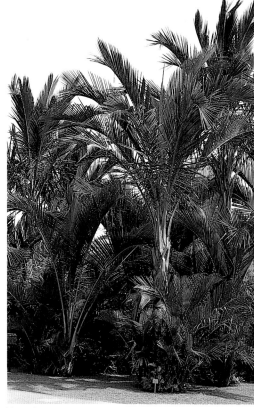

Metroxylon sagu

rots away, and is replaced by the suckers, or young palms. The stem of a matured palm is filled with starch in its soft centre. By felling the palm just before flowering, the maximum amount of sago can be extracted.

Parts used:
fruits: disperse superficial blood clots
sago: nutritive and strengthening

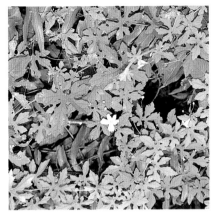

Momordica charantia

MOMORDICA
FAMILY: Cucurbitaceae
Momordica
momordica

This is a vine of the Old World tropics. The generic name, *Momordica* is Latin, "to bite", in reference to the seeds, the edge of which appears as if bitten.

Momordica charantia 苦瓜
bitter gourd
balsam pear
bitter cucumber
la gua
The plant is grown for the bitter fruits which are eaten as a vegetable in India and the Far East. Originating from the Old World, it is now widely spread in the tropics.

Parts used:
fruit: cools the body system; purgative; tonic; treats fever

Momordica cochinchinensis 木鱉子
Parts used:
seeds: treat chest complaints, liver and spleen disorders, piles, malaria, wounds, bruises, swellings

MORINDA
FAMILY: Rubiaceae
Morinda
morinda
menkudu

Morindas are tropical plants, with fleshy, oval fruits developing from the flowering head. Fruits are edible but tend to be unsavoury when ripe, often with a rancid smell as well. These plants provide a yellow dye called morindin, obtained from the roots. The dye was once used extensively on native cloth, especially in the Javanese *batik* industry, to give red, purple and pink shades.

Morinda citrifolia 橘叶巴戟
great morinda
Indian mulberry
The plant is found from China to Southeast Asia. It is commonly used in the native medicines of the region.

Parts used:
whole plant: treats aching bones

Morinda officinalis 巴戟天
Chinese morinda
The plant is found wild in China as well as under cultivation. The fleshy roots are collected from plants at least five years old and used medicinally.

Parts used:
roots: tonic in the treatment of beriberi; strengthen the kidneys; increase menstrual flow; treat tendon and bone ailments, premature ejaculation, impotence, female infertility, lumbago, hernia, excessive or involuntary discharge of urine

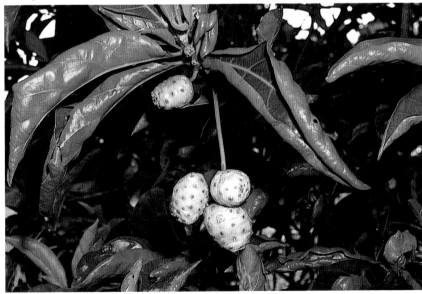

Morinda citrifolia

MORUS
FAMILY: Moraceae
Morus alba 桑
white mulberry

This is a wide-spreading tree with a rounded crown, thick trunk and heart-shaped leaves. It is native to China, Indochina, Japan and the Philippines. The trees are often planted for the edible fruit, and the leaves of a specific variety are used for silkworm culture. The figs can be made into jams and jellies or fermented to yield an alcohol. The bark gives a fibre, used in weaving.

Parts used:
leaves: treat fever, cold, cough, conjunctivitis
skin of the roots: expels phlegm from the respiratory system in asthma; treats bronchitis, coughs
figs: tonic; treat insomnia, high blood pressure

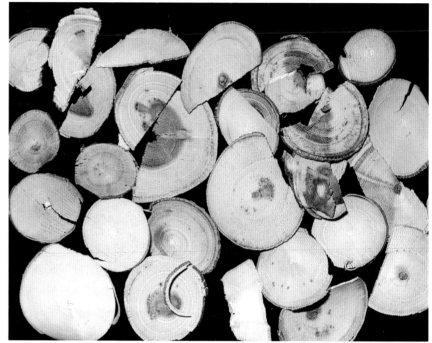

Morus alba

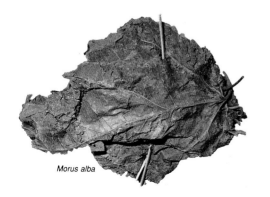

Morus alba

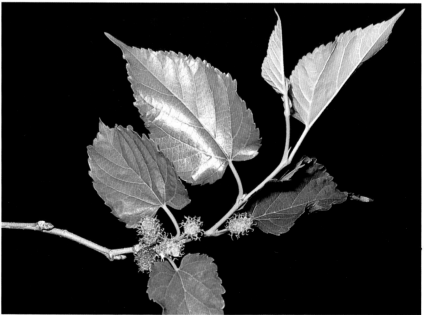

Morus

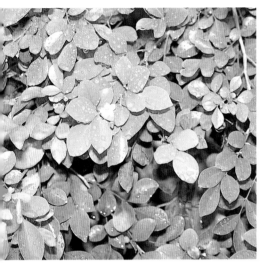

va paniculata

MURRAYA
FAMILY: Rutaceae
Murraya paniculata 九里香
mock orange
orange jasmine
Chinese box

The plant is named in honour of
J. A. Myrray (1740–1791), editor
of Linnaeus' *Systema
Vegetabilium*. The rather small
tree is very attractive due to the
glossy leaves, and cultivated
widely in the tropics as an
ornament. Native to Southeast
Asia, it has compound leaves
and fragrant, white flowers.
Fruits are ovoid and red.

Parts used:
leaves: relieve pain; treat
stomachache, chronic dysentery,
bruises, swellings, itching, skin
irritation

MYRISTICA
FAMILY: Myristicaceae
Myristica fragrans 肉豆蔻
nutmeg

The generic name, *Myristica*, is
derived from a medieval word
for nut, meaning "suitable for an
ointment". The specific name,
fragrans, refers to the fragrance
of the plant. The medium-sized
tree bears small, pale yellow,
inconspicuous flowers, the male
flowers on different trees from
the female. However,
occasionally, both types of
flowers may be found on the
same tree. Fruits are roundish,
yellow and fleshy; they split into
two at maturity to expose the
jet-black seed covered with a
lacy red, membranous mace. A
native of the Moluccas, the trees
are grown commercially in
Indonesia and the West Indian
island of Grenada for the seed
and mace.

The seed is added to the
quid by betel chewers for
intoxicating effects. Powdered,
the seed or mace is sniffed or
taken orally to get high,
accompanied by hallucinations.
If taken in excess, it can be
toxic. The toxic and narcotic
properties are due to the
presence of myristicin; in small
amounts they may improve
appetite as well as promote
digestion. It is also claimed to
have aphrodisiac and abortive
properties.

The dried seed is used grated
to flavour cakes, punches and
milk dishes. Mace is used with
savoury dishes, and in pickles
and ketchups. The husk of the
fruit is made into sweetmeats in
Malaysia. The seed also gives
nutmeg butter, used in
ointments and perfumes. Oil of
nutmeg, obtained by distillation,
is used in medicine and
perfumery.

In 17th century Europe,
nutmegs encased in silver were
worn at night to induce sleep.
Because the fruit is believed to
have aphrodisiac properties, it
has always been a standard
ingredient in love potions.

Parts used:
seed: removes excessive gas in
the system; treats indigestion,
muscle spasms, heart diseases,
diarrhoea, rheumatism
flowers, mace, seeds, oil: treat
excessive discharge of fluids
from the body (such as watery
faeces), stomach cramps, heart
diseases, chronic rheumatism

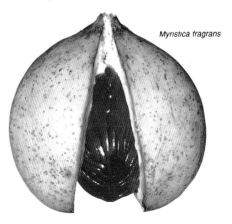

Myristica fragrans

123

NARDOSTACHYS
FAMILY: Valerianaceae
Nardostachys

These are erect herbs with woody underground stems and fragrant roots. They are native to the high alpine meadows of the Himalayas and China.

Nardostachys chinensis 甘松香
The underground stems are collected and left unwashed, as washing would remove the fragrance. They are sweet and warming, and used to treat various ailments.

Parts used:
underground stem: treats toothache, congested chest and stomach; relieves pain; bath for a swollen ankle to relieve pain and bring down swelling

Nardostachys jatamansi 宽叶甘松
The underground stems yield the aromatic ointment, spikenard, used by the ancients.

Parts used:
underground stems: stimulant; deodorant; nerve tonic; treat skin problems, headache, colic, mental depression

NELUMBO
FAMILY: Nymphaeaceae
Nelumbo nucifera 莲
lotus
sacred lotus
East Indian lotus

The generic name is of Sri Lankan origin. This large, attractive plant of freshwater ponds and lakes is often cultivated for the edible stem and seeds. It is native to countries from South Asia to Australia. The leaves are up to 1 m across, usually rising above the surface of the water on stout stalks. The flowers are fragrant and variously coloured: pink, rose or sometimes white. The more than 20 seeds, which are embedded in the flat surface of the spongy triangular receptacle of the flower, are edible. They are detached by hand and their tiny embryo removed before being eaten raw or cooked in a number of ways. A number of cultivars are in existence, differentiated by the flowers.

In Asia, the lotus has taken a deep symbolic meaning. The Indians regard it as an embodiment of female serenity and a symbol of eternal reproduction. The Japanese on the other hand associate it with death, the flower being a standard offering at funerals. The flower is also sacred to the Buddhists.

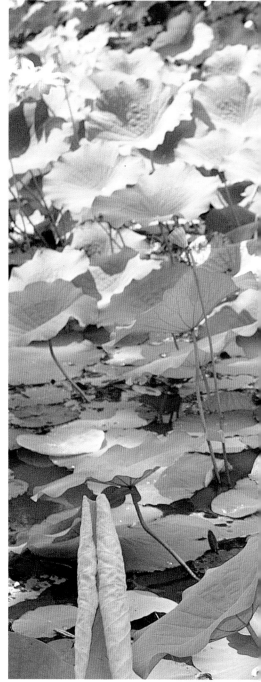

Nelumbo nucifera

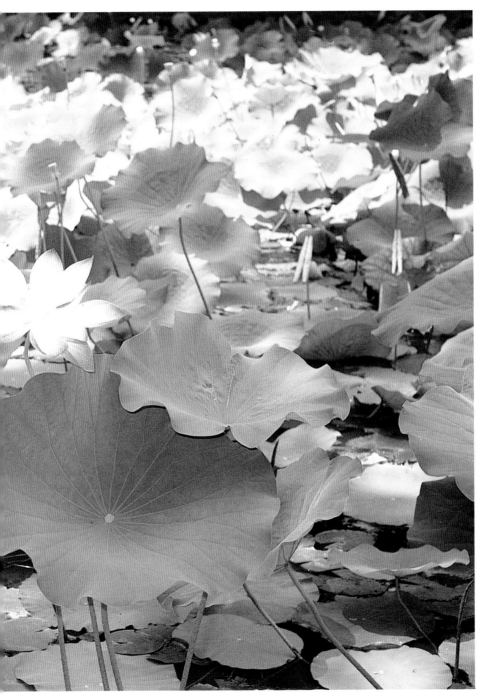

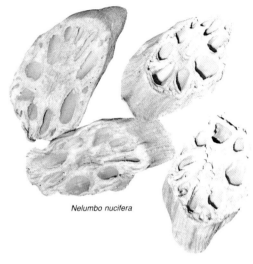

Nelumbo nucifera

Parts used:
whole plant: antidote for mushroom poisoning
leaves: treat sunstroke, diarrhoea, dysentery, fever, dizziness, vomiting of blood
flower stalks: treat excessive bleeding from the uterus
flowers: treat premature ejaculation
seeds: tonic

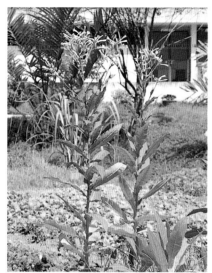
Nicotiana tabacum

NICOTIANA
FAMILY: Solanaceae
Nicotiana tabacum 烟草
tobacco

The generic name, *Nicotiana*, commemorates Jean Nicot (1530–1600), the French consul to Portugal who, it was said, was the first person to present tobacco to the courts of Portugal and France. The specific name, *tabacum*, is the Latinized version of an American aboriginal name, from which also comes the word tobacco. Some people believe that it is derived from the Haitian word for the pipe in which tobacco is smoked; the plant originated from tropical America. It has been cultivated by the American Indians since ancient times, and now is cultivated widely for the cigarette and cigar industries.

The use of tobacco was observed by Columbus in the West Indies in 1492. The plant was introduced into Europe where it was grown as an ornament and used medicinally. It was only towards the end of the 16th century that the habit of smoking became widespread in Europe. By the 17th century the habit had spread to Asia and Africa. Now the use of tobacco is seen throughout the world, whether chewed, smoked or snuffed. Despite heavy taxes imposed by most governments, providing considerable revenues, the habit persists.

Parts used:
plant: treats soreness of the joints, numbness, rheumatism, snake bites

OCIMUM
FAMILY: Labiatae
Ocimum basilicum 罗勒
common basil
sweet basil

Basils are aromatic plants so aptly implied in the generic name, *Ocimum*, which comes from the Greek word, *osme*, meaning "smell". The common name, basil, comes from the Greek *basilicon*, "royal". The ancient Greeks associated the plant with hatred and abusive language and abused the seeds prior to sowing them to ensure satisfactory growth. Common basil is a hairy annual herb, native to the Old World tropics. The plant is commonly grown for the fragrant foliage, used as a flavouring in cooking. It yields camphor of basil, used in perfumery and liquor distillery.

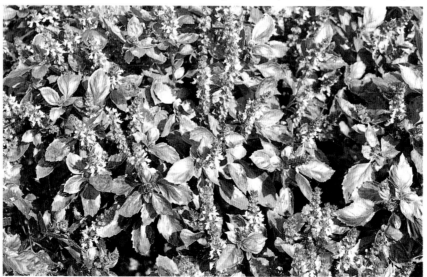
Ocimum basilicum

The camphor can also be used as a mosquito repellent.

Parts used:
leaves: tonic; treat excessive gas in the system, vomiting, hiccups

OPHIOPOGON
FAMILY: Liliaceae
Ophiopogon japonicus 沿阶草
dwarf lilyturf
mondo grass

The plant is an evergreen, stemless herb, native to Japan and Korea. It is cultivated in eastern and western China. The dried tuberous roots, with the inner fibrous portion removed, are used medicinally, either treated or untreated with mercuric oxide.

Parts used:
roots: cool the body system; tonic; purgative; thirst quencher; treat sore throat, cough, fever

OROXYLUM
FAMILY: Bignoniaceae
Oroxylum indicum 木蝴蝶
midnight horror

The midnight horror is a large evergreen tree reaching 20 m tall, with sparse branching and large compound leaves of 1 to 2 m in length, looking like branches themselves. Leaves are crowded at the ends of branches and, when they wither, the leaflets fall off, followed by the side stalks and main stalks. These stalks accumulate at the base of the

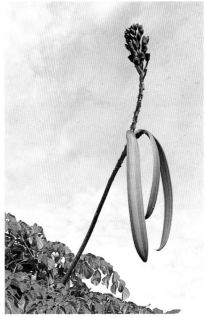
Oroxylum indicum

tree like a collection of bones, thus its other name, broken bone plant. The large flowers are in terminal bunches, the buds filled with a liquid. They open at night, emitting a powerful stink to attract bats which help in the pollination. Fruits are long, flat pods, filled with large flat seeds, surrounded by a thin, transparent wing. The tree is native to Asia, from the foot of the Himalayas and southern China to India and parts of Southeast Asia.

Parts used:
seeds: treat throat infection, coughs, abdominal pain, mouth ulcers

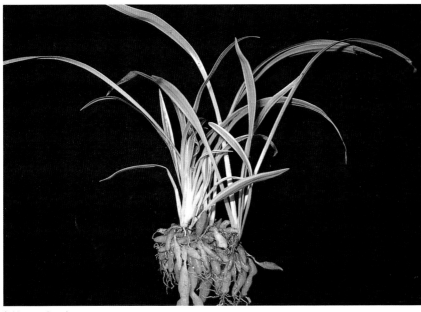
Ophiopogon japonicus

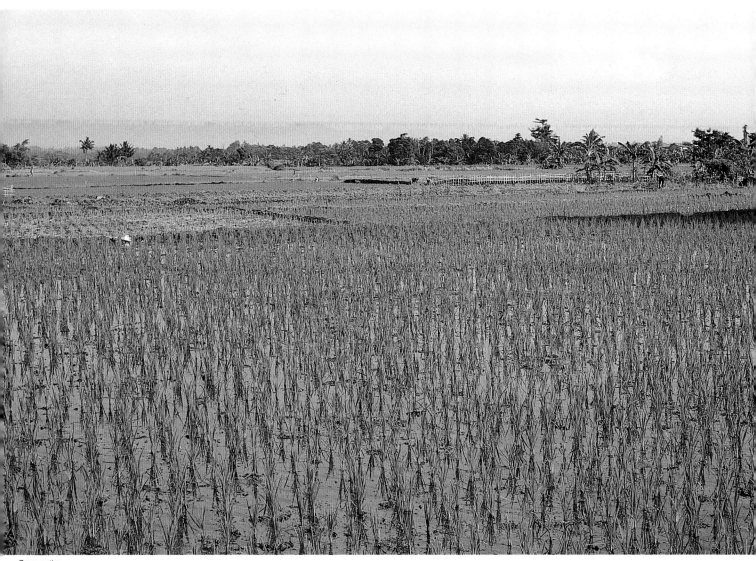

Oryza sativa

ORYZA
FAMILY: Gramineae

Oryza sativa 稲
rice

The generic name for rice is an adaptation of the Arabic name, *eruz*. The plant is an annual, standing about 1 m tall and consisting of conspicuously elongated leaves. The flowering shoot consists of numerous individual units bearing the floral parts, which are never showy. Fruits, oblong and yellowish white, are found inside the brown husk.

Rice is one of the most important economic crop, providing food for half the world's population. It has been in cultivation in Southeast Asia since ancient times, being commonly cultivated in fresh water swampy areas, although dry-land rice also exists and is grown in hilly areas. The plant was probably domesticated in India or Indochina about 5000 years ago but definite evidence is lacking. Through selection and hybridization, thousands of cultivars exist today. Rice plays an important role in many religious and magical rites in the East, its significance being variously related to fecundity and plenty. It is believed that the western custom of throwing rice at weddings originates from an ancient eastern fertility cult.

Parts used:
germinating grains: tonic; treat gastric problems
rice water: cools the body system; treats nose bleed

OXALIS
FAMILY: Oxalidaceae
Oxalis corniculata 酢浆草
yellow wood sorrel

The generic name is derived from the Greek *oxys*, "sharp" or "acid", referring to the acidity of the leaves. Some people claim that the "triple leaf" of the wood sorrel is the true shamrock of St Patrick, the national emblem of Ireland. According to legend, St Patrick used the wood sorrel leaf to explain the Holy Trinity to his pagan audience in Ireland when trying to convert them to Christianity. This cosmopolitan weed is a creeping herbaceous plant of grassy areas and wastelands.

Parts used:
plant: cooling agent; expels intestinal worms; increases flow of urine, controls bleeding

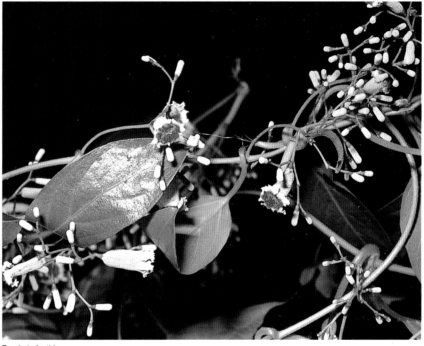
Paederia foetida

PAEDERIA
FAMILY: Rubiaceae
Paederia foetida 鸡矢藤
stinkwort
akar sekentut
daun kentut-kentut

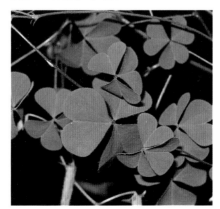
Oxalis corniculata

As the common name implies, the plant has a characteristic stink when the leaves are crushed. The Malay names have similar connotation. Even its scientific name has reference to the foetid smell the leaves emit. The plant is a weedy scrambler of open spaces in India, China, the Philippines and Peninsular Malaysia.

Parts used:
leaves: help in digestion; expel gas; remedy for poisonous insect bites

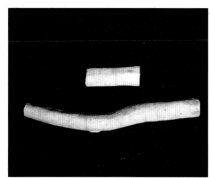
Paeonia lactiflora

PAEONIA
FAMILY: Ranunculaceae
Paeonia
peony

These are shrubs or herbs, native to north temperate Eurasia and western North America. They are among the most popular garden plants as they bear colourful flowers. Peony or the genus *Paeonia* is named after the Greek physician, Paeon, who was the first in the western world to use the plant for medicinal purposes. The ancient Greeks believed the plant to be of divine origin, coming from the moon, and thus having the power to shine at night.

During the Victorian period, English children wore necklaces made from this plant to help their teething and prevent convulsions. Elizabethan children similarly used necklaces made from seeds of peony to keep witches at bay. As the plant had the reputation of keeping away evil spirits, it was planted near houses. Seeds were taken at night and in the morning to prevent nightmares. Old English herbalists used the roots to cleanse the womb after childbirth.

Paeonia lactiflora 芍药
Chinese peony
Native to China, Korea, Manchuria, Siberia and Japan, the plant is commonly cultivated for the attractive flowers as well as for medicinal purposes. Hundreds of cultivars have been derived from this species.

Parts used:
roots: intestinal antiseptic; promote the expulsion of phlegm; increase menstrual flow; increase flow of urine; treat cholera, tuberculosis, general weakness, vomiting, stomach problems

Paeonia suffruticosa 牡丹
tree peony
This is a coarsely branched shrub with white to rose-pink flowers. It is native to the region from Bhutan to Tibet and China.

Parts used:
root bark: treats fever-induced vomiting of blood, scarlet fever, convulsions, bleeding; induces menstruation

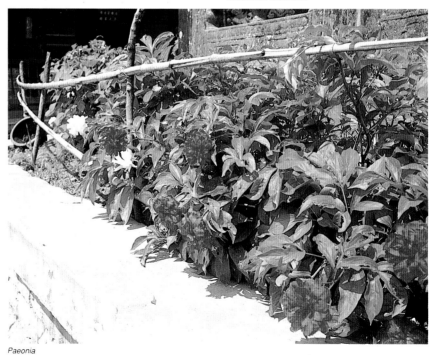
Paeonia

PANAX

FAMILY: Araliaceae

Panax pseudoginseng 三七
Asiatic ginseng
Panax ginseng 人参
ginseng

This plant is considered a panacea, as seen in its generic name which comes from the Greek word *Panakes*, meaning "a panacea", or "all healing". The herb is native to Manchuria and Korea and cultivated in Japan. Flowers are small, yellow-green and in terminal heads. Fruits are small, red berries. The fleshy underground roots are aromatic and often divided at the ends.

Many legends surround this plant. One has it that during the Sui dynasty, the nightly wailing of a man was subsequently traced to a plant, the roots of which resembled the figure of a man. Another claimed that ginseng hunters sought out the plants under the cover of darkness, spotting them by the phosphorescent glow of the flowers. They then aimed an arrow at the glow to mark the spot, as the slightest sound caused the flowers to close and the glow to go off. The next morning the arrow was located and the roots dug out.

The Chinese have long regarded the roots of ginseng as a panacea, mainly because of their resemblance to the human

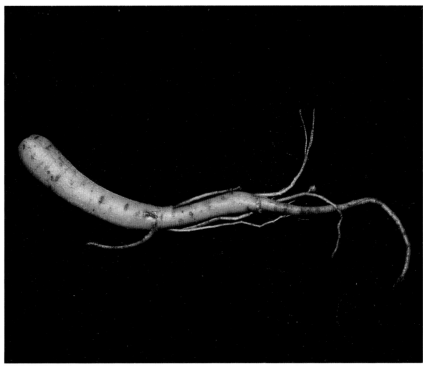

Panax pseudoginseng

form. Ginseng roots are available today in various forms: they are powdered, preserved in alcohol, sliced, and in concentrated extracts, tincture, wholes, tea bags or capsules.

Extensive research has been conducted during the last four decades to unveil the secrets of the roots. Several physiologically active substances have since been isolated: panaxin, panax acid, panaquilon, panacen, sapogenin and ginsenin. The last has been shown to be beneficial against diabetes. Japanese scientists have isolated a substance called ginsenocide, from the red ginseng plant. This substance is claimed to arrest the growth of cancer cells in tests with white mice. So far researchers have yet to test it on humans.

Parts used:
roots: tonic; sedative; stimulant; aphrodisiac; treat anaemia, general weakness after vomiting blood, nervous disorders, shortness of breath, perspiration, forgetfulness, excessive menstrual bleeding, impotence, fever, excessive sweating, thirst

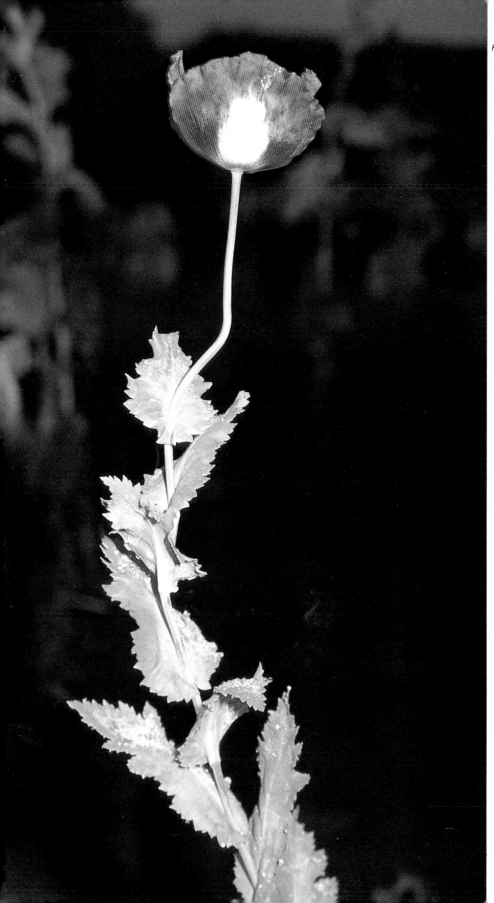

PAPAVER
FAMILY: Papaveraceae
Papaver somniferum 罌粟
opium poppy

Opium poppy is a strong smelling, low herb, native to southeastern Europe and West Asia. The plant bears attractive flowers which are white, red, purple or pink. These develop into roundish capsules with terminal pores, from which the many small seeds are shaken out. The generic name, *Papaver*, is the Latin word for poppy while the specific name, *somniferum*, means sleep-producing. Opium is Latin *opium*, derived from the Greek word *opion*, meaning "opium" or "poppy juice". In Roman mythology the poppy is associated with Somnus, god of sleep. Somnus was said to have created the plant for Ceres, the goddess of harvest, to enable her to rest as she was neglecting the crops due to tiredness. According to Greek mythology the flower is associated with Hypnus, god of sleep.

Opium is obtained by making incisions on the surface of the young, developing fruit. The sap oozes out and, when partially dried, is scraped and collected into cakes and dried in the sun. The resulting blackish mass is opium. The most important constituents of opium are the alkaloids, with morphine being the main one. The drug was known since ancient times, used chiefly in medicine as a hypnotic and sedative. It was administered to relieve pain and to calm an excited person.

Parts used:
empty fruits: treat coughs, spasms, headache, toothache, asthma, diarrhoea
opium: used for its narcotic, antispasmodic, sedative, analgesic and hypnotic properties

PAULOWNIA
FAMILY: Scrophulariaceae
Paulownia tomentosa 毛泡桐
princess tree

This is a deciduous tree, native to China. The tree has large, hairy leaves which vary from unlobed to three-lobed. It reaches a height of 20 m. The fragrant flowers are pale violet with darker spots inside. The generic name commemorates Anna Paulownia (1795–1865), princess of the Netherlands.

Parts used:
bark, wood: expel intestinal worms; treat ulcers, falling hairs, delirium as a result of typhoid fever
leaves: promote growth of hair; restore colour to hair; treat sores

PERILLA
FAMILY: Labiatae
Perilla frutescens var. *crispa* 皱紫苏
perilla

This is an erect annual herb found in southern China, Taiwan, Japan, northern Vietnam, Laos, Thailand, India and Burma. It is widely cultivated for the seeds from which an oil is obtained.

Parts used:
leaves, seeds: stimulate gastric activities; treat coughs, influenza, nausea during pregnancy

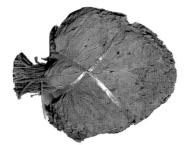

Perilla frutescens

PHELLODENDRON
FAMILY: Rutaceae
Phellodendron amurense 黄柏
Amur cork tree

The generic name, *Phellodendron,* comes from the Greek words *phellos* meaning "cork" and *dendron* "tree", in reference to the bark of the original cork tree. The specific name *amurense* comes from Amur, a river in northeastern

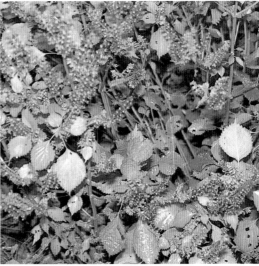

Perilla frutescens

Asia, which forms the boundary between Manchuria and the Soviet Union, probably the location where the first plant was seen. This tall deciduous tree from northern China, Siberia and Japan is a popular ornamental tree because of its orange-yellow branchlets and deeply fissured, corky bark. The flowers are yellow-green and smell of turpentine when bruised. The plant is used for almost every ailment known to the Chinese, and is known as a poor man's "cure all".

Parts used:
bark: treats dysentery, sweating at night, blood in the urine, kidney problems, lumbago, jaundice, yellowish discharge from vagina, vaginal itching, dermatitis

133

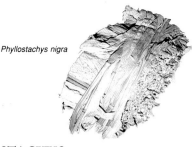
Phyllostachys nigra

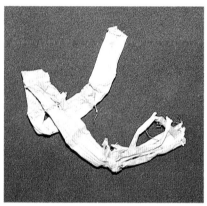
Phragmites

PHRAGMITES
Family: Gramineae
Phragmites australis 芦苇
reed grass

The generic name, *Phragmites*, is derived from the Greek word *phragma*, meaning "materials for an enclosure", as the long stems of the reed grass were widely used in thatching house roofs and barns.
According to Greek mythology, the Titan Prometheus stole fire from Olympus and brought it to mankind in a hollow reed. For his troubles he was chained to a rock where an eagle tore at his liver until Hercules freed him. This rather tall grass of marshy areas has a creeping rootstock from which arise the erect shoots. The flowering shoot develops from the top of the vegetative shoot, consisting of compact, purplish brown or reddish flowers. This grass is of worldwide distribution.

Parts used:
underground stems, roots: treat cough with yellow sputum, pain in the lungs, stomach fever, vomiting, hiccups

PHYLLANTHUS
FAMILY: Euphorbiaceae
Phyllanthus emblica 油柑
Malacca tree
emblic
Melaka
asam Melaka
laka laka

The tree is Southeast Asian in origin, growing in villages and in lowland forests. The fruits are round and juicy, rather sour, and eaten as a relish.

Parts used:
roots: purgative

PHYLLOSTACHYS
FAMILY: Gramineae
Phyllostachys nigra 紫竹
black bamboo

The generic name is Greek, meaning "leaf-spike". The plant is native to China but has been in cultivation for a long time in Japan as well as in Europe and elsewhere as an ornament. The tall (3–10 m) evergreen bamboo has a 3 cm diameter stem which is green at first, slowly turning brown then purple-black. The joints of the stem are prominent, being blackish on the upper rim and white on the lower.

Parts used:
leaves: encourage flow of urine; suppress fever
roots: check blood flow; restrict secretions of body fluids
stem shavings: sedative; suppress vomiting; treat fever

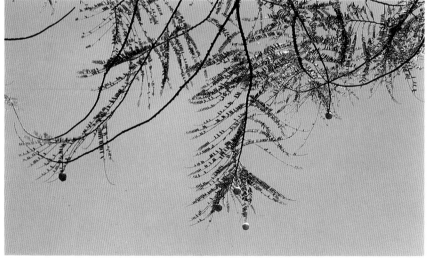
Phyllanthus emblica

tachys nigra

クロチク

16クロチク

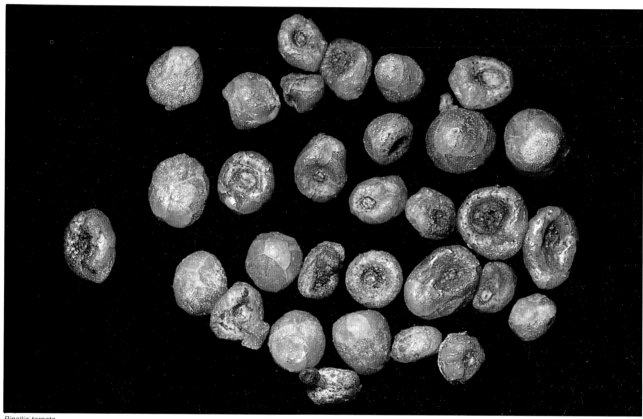

Pinellia ternata

PINELLIA
FAMILY: Araceae
Pinellia ternata 半夏
pinellia

The plant is commonly cultivated in fields and by roadsides in southern China, Korea and Japan. It grows from an underground stem, bearing leaves with three leaflets; each leaflet has a small bulb-like swelling at the middle and the uppermost part of the leaf stalk. Flowers are small and inconspicuous, and develop into green fruits. The raw underground stem is poisonous and needs special processing for use internally. Before being used, in Chinese medicine, the pieces are first bleached with sulphur fumes, soaked in water and boiled with alum, then dried. Thus prepared, the pieces appear white to yellowish white, with a pure white interior. Alternatively, pieces are boiled with ginger and then with alum, dried and pounded into a powder. The underground stem has been used as an anticancer remedy in other folk medicine; this activity has been confirmed in experiments with animals.

Parts used:
underground stem: causes sweating; increases flow of urine; treats nausea during pregnancy, inflammation of the liver, vomiting, chronic kidney disease, skin diseases, blisters, abscesses, ulcers

PINUS
FAMILY: Pinaceae
Pinus
pine

Pines are tall coniferous trees, native to the northern hemisphere. Many are important timber trees. Leaves are aromatic and of two kinds: scale-like and needlelike. The latter are long and in clusters of twos. The male cones are collected, dried and rubbed between the hands to release the sweet pollen, which is used to increase blood cells.

Pinus massoniana 马尾松
Pinus tabuliformis 油松
These trees are native to China where they are important timber trees.

Parts used:
pollen: relieve headache; sprinkled on boils to dry up pus
pine knots: treat rheumatism, toothache

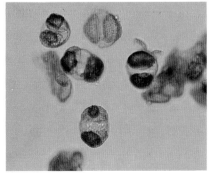

Pinus

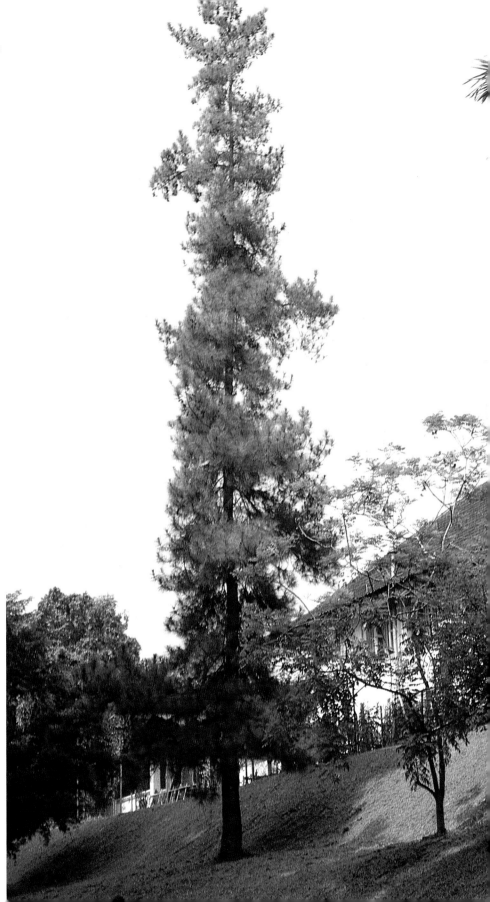

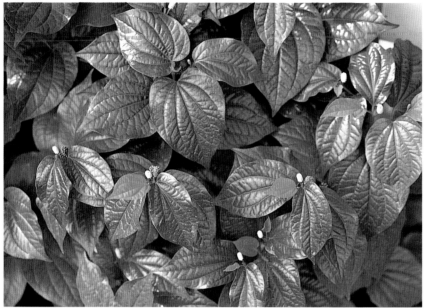

Piper sarmentosum

PIPER
FAMILY: Piperaceae

Piper
pepper

These are shrubs, treelike or even climbing plants of tropical distribution. The plant has a characteristic pungent odour and swollen joints.

Piper nigrum 胡椒
pepper plant
black pepper
white pepper

This is a vine with a stout stem bearing short climbing roots. There are separate plants bearing male and female flowers. Fruits are rounded and turn from green to red. Native to southern India and Sri Lanka, pepper is widely planted throughout the tropics especially in the West Indies and Brazil, for the berries which are highly valued as a spice. Dried unripe fruits provide the black pepper of commerce while white pepper is obtained by removing the skins.

Parts used:
fruits: remove excessive gas in the system; increase flow of urine; treat colic, rheumatism, headache, diarrhoea, dysentery, cholera, menstrual pains

Piper sarmentosum 假蒟
This plant is found in India, southern China and Indonesia.

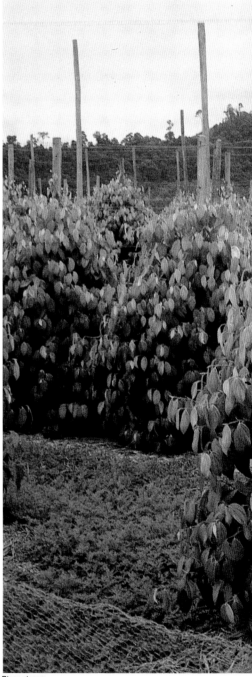

Piper nigrum

138

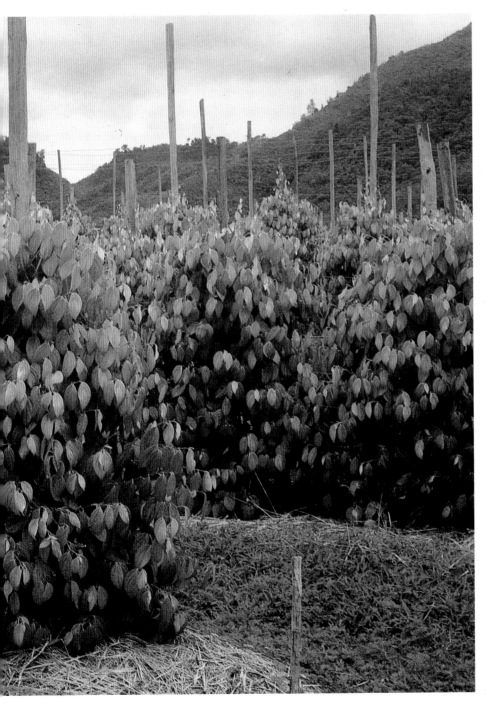

Parts used:
whole plant: treats fever; aids digestion
roots: treat toothache

Piper cubeba 荜澄茄
Parts used:
fruits: remove excessive gas from the system; treat vomiting, stomach disorders, sunstroke

PISTIA
FAMILY: Araceae
Pistia stratiotes 水浮莲
water lettuce

The generic name comes from the Greek *pistos*, in reference to its aquatic habitat. This is a floating, stemless herb found commonly in stagnant waters throughout the tropics and the subtropics.

Parts used:
whole plant: increases menstrual flow; treats skin complaints

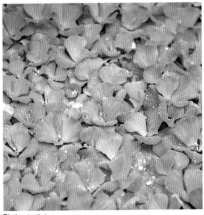

Pistia stratiotes

139

PLANTAGO
FAMILY: Plantaginaceae
Plantago major 车前
common plantain
white-man's foot
cart-track plant

This herb is native to northern and central Asia as well as to Europe. It is now a weed in many parts of the world. The generic name may have been derived from the Latin *planta*, meaning "the sole of the foot", in allusion to the shape of the leaves as they lie on the ground. The plant is commonly known as white-man's foot by the American Indians as they believe that the plant was introduced by the early settlers, who arrive from Europe with the seeds in their pockets and their shoes. The watery extracts of the plant are used in cosmetics and the stem and seeds as bird food.

The plant is used in homeopathy for toothache, middle ear disease, involuntary discharge of urine, abnormally fast beating of the heart and healing of wounds and sores. In orthodox medicine the plant is administered internally to treat bleeding, coughing of blood, bleeding following childbirth, inflammation of the mucus membrane of the lungs; and the seeds used as purgative, to suppress urine, and to treat haemorrhagic diarrhoea, dysentery and coughs.

The seed coat of most *Plantago* species contains a high content of mucilage, thus it has a soothing effect if applied externally, or internally in the case of treating coughs.

Parts used:
seeds: induce sweating; increase flow of urine; treat diarrhoea, dysentery, rheumatism, malaria, asthma, kidney problems, bladder diseases, gonorrhoea, piles

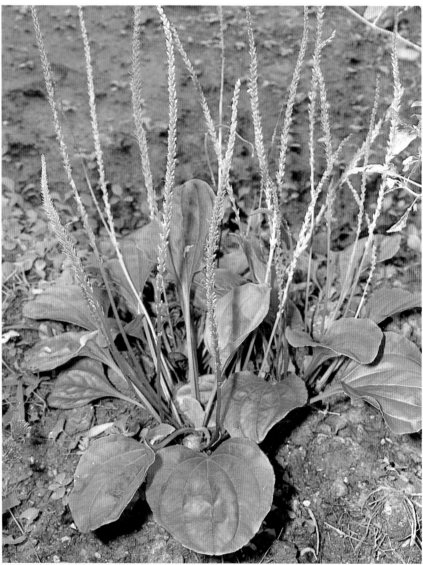
Plantago major

PLATYCLADUS
FAMILY: Cupressaceae
Platycladus orientalis 侧柏
oriental arbor-vitae

The plant is a medium-sized, aromatic, evergreen tree, native to China and Korea. The shape of the tree and the branchlets, arranged in a vertical plane, make it a rather attractive tree for ornamental planting. The leaves are reduced to scales that are arranged along the stem in two pairs of opposite rows so as to totally cover its entire length. The female cones are oval and 2.5 cm long, and contain thick seeds which are wingless. In Singapore the tree is grown in gardens but they do not bear cones. In homeopathy the leaves, in the form of a tincture, are used to treat warts and swellings of the mucus membrane.

Parts used:
seeds: sedative in the treatment of minor headache; treat insomnia, heart palpitation
leaves: increase menstrual flow; treat fever, nose bleeds, vomiting of blood, blood in the urine

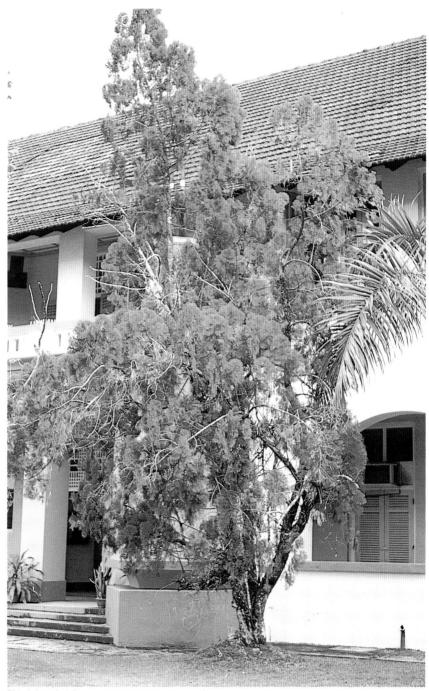

Platycladus orientalis

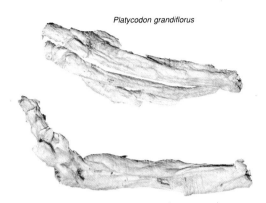

Platycodon grandiflorus

PLATYCODON
FAMILY: Campanulaceae
Platycodon grandiflorus 桔梗
Chinese bell flower
balloon flower

The name "balloon flower" comes from the inflated flower buds, looking like balloons or bells. The generic name, in Greek, means "broad bell" and the specific name means "large flower". This erect shrub with red stem comes from China and Japan. It is commonly cultivated and a number of cultivars are in existence. The flowers are large and showy, ranging from dark to pale blue, to white, and usually solitary, on a long stalk.

Parts used:
roots: stomach tonic for indigestion; remove excessive gas in the system; expel intestinal worms; treat stomach ulcers, dysentery, cholera, influenza, sore throat, asthma, colds, nausea, chest congestion, tonsillitis

PLUMERIA
FAMILY: Apocynaceae
Plumeria rubra 鸡蛋花
frangipani

The common name, frangipani, honours the Marquis Muzio Frangipani, a 16th century Roman nobleman who invented the perfume for scenting gloves. The genus, *Plumeria*, on the other hand, is named after C. Plumier, a French botanist (1646–1706). These medium-sized trees are native to tropical America, now planted widely throughout the tropics. Branching is sparse and the sticky white latex mildly poisonous. A number of species are recognized, together with many hybrids, a result of years of breeding and selection. The flowers are large, fragrant and showy, in white, yellow, pink or red. Fruits are twin pods containing numerous flat, shortly winged seeds.

Frangipani trees are commonly planted in gardens and parks of warm countries. To the Buddhists, Hindus and Muslims, the tree signifies immortality because it continues to produce flowers and leaves even after it has been uprooted. For this reason the tree is often planted near Buddhist and Hindu temples. Muslims plant the tree in graveyards as the daily fall of flowers are taken as fresh floral offerings to the dead. The planting of a tree by a grave in Peninsular Malaysia is a Malay custom, probably originating from Hindu influences.

Parts used:
flowers: treat diarrhoea, cough, dysentery

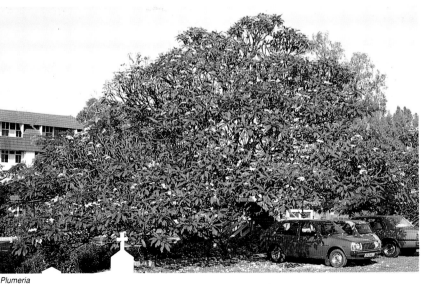

Plumeria

POGOSTEMON
FAMILY: Labiatae
Pogostemon cablin 广藿香
patchouli

This is a very fragrant plant, once grown for the leaves which were used to distill a fragrant oil used in perfumery. The plant is native to Southeast Asia and probably introduced by overseas Chinese into China as a medicinal plant. It has been used medicinally in China for more than a hundred years.

Parts used:
whole plant: treats headache, gas in the system, vomiting, diarrhoea

POLYGALA
FAMILY: Polygalaceae
Polygala
milkwort

Milkworts are trees, shrubs and herbs found widely around the world. The generic name, *Polygala*, comes from the Greek words, *polys* and *gala*, for "much milk", as there is an ancient belief that the plant increases the flow of milk in animals.

Polygala tenuifolia 细叶远志
This is a tall shrub, native to northern China and Mongolia.

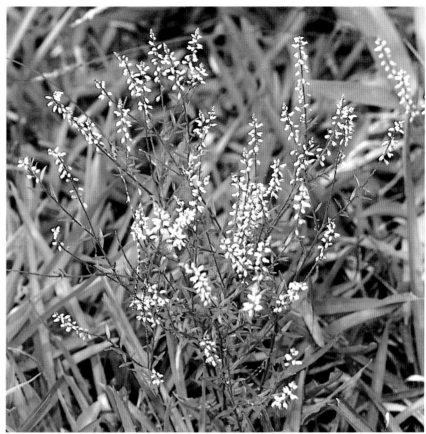
Polygala

Parts used:
roots: expel phlegm from respiratory passages; treat coughs, swellings, heart palpitation, insomnia, amnesia, jaundice, hysteria, abscesses of the heart

Polygala telephoides 小花远志
Parts used:
whole plant: dissolves blood clots; treats shortness of breath, opium poisoning

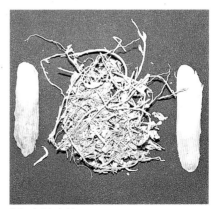
Polygala telephoides

143

POLYGONATUM

FAMILY: Liliaceae

Polygonatum
Solomon's seal
King Solomon's seal

These plants are native to temperate North America, Europe and Asia. They have an underground stem which is much jointed, with scars all over. Flowers are greenish to yellow, developing into blue-black or red berries. The generic name comes from the Greek words, *polys* and *gony*, meaning "many knees", in reference to the jointed underground stem of the plant. The origin of the common names is not clear. There are those who believe that the hanging flowers suggest a bunch of seals; or that the round, flat scars on the underground stem resemble a Solomon's seal, a name given by Arabs to a six-pointed star. Others believe that, as the flower stems decay, the scars on the main stalk resemble seals, or that the roots have the properties to heal (or seal) wounds.

The plants are poisonous and there have been cases in which children are poisoned as a result of eating the sweetish berries. They contain saponins, and some people believe that there are cardiac glycosides as well. European folk medicine uses the underground stem to make a tea to treat diabetes. Japanese folk medicine uses the stem for diabetes as well.

Polygonatum cirrhifolium 卷叶黄精
This is native to northern China and the Himalayas.

Parts used:
rootstock: tonic; treats rheumatism, bruises

Polygonatum odoratum 玉竹
This is a widely cultivated plant in China and Japan. The underground stem is sweet and cooling.

Parts used:
underground stem: tonic; thirst quencher; treats lung fever, hacking cough, common cold, sore throat, weakness after illness, rheumatism

POLYGONUM

FAMILY: Polygonaceae

Polygonum
knotweed

The generic name comes from the Greek words, *polys* and *gony*, meaning "many knees", in reference to the jointed stems of these plants. Almost all knotweeds have stems which are jointed, and therefore, brittle. Thus the stems snap easily when collected. The jointed stems also give these plants a characteristic appearance. Knotweeds are herbs of wide distribution. Many are weeds of arable land, roadsides and wastelands. A few are of ornamental value, as their many small, white, green or red flowers are rather attractive. Many are also of medicinal value, commonly used among European as well as oriental herbalists.

In Chinese medicine a number of species are used, all of which are found in China.

Polygonum aviculare 萹蓄
Parts used:
plant: alleviates pain during urination; treats blood in the urine, gonorrhoea, diarrhoea, jaundice, roundworm infection, stones in the kidney and bladder, bleeding in ulcers

Polygonum chinense 火炭母草
Parts used:
plant: purifies blood; treats dysentery, headache
roots: expel intestinal worms

Polygonum cuspidatum 虎杖
Japanese knotweed
Mexican bamboo

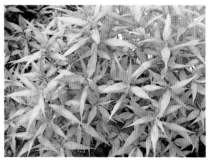

Polygonum hydropiper

144

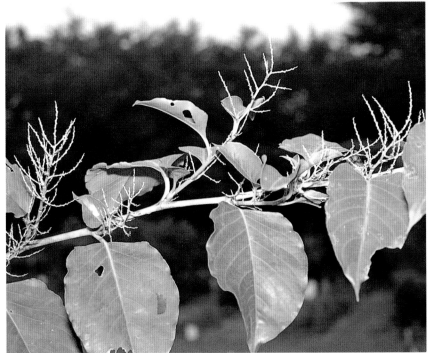

Polygonum cuspidatum

Parts used:
roots: treat gout, rheumatoid arthritis, jaundice, gonorrhoea

Polygonum hydropiper 水蓼
Parts used:
whole plant: treat diarrhoea, dysentery, itching of the skin

Polygonum multiflorum 何首乌
Parts used:
roots: treat dizziness, tuberculosis of the lymphatic glands, cancer, constipation, insomnia

Polygonum orientale 红蓼
prince's-feather
princess-feather
kiss-me-over-the-garden-gate

The plant, a hairy herb, is native to Asia and Australia. It has bright pink or rose flowers.

Parts used:
fruits: treat general inflammation, inflammation of the liver

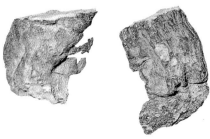

Polygonum multiflorum

PRUNELLA
FAMILY: Labiatae
Prunella vulgaris 夏枯草
heal-all
self-heal

The generic name of this plant is said to be from the German *braune*, a disease of the throat, for which the plant was a remedy. As the common name implies, the heal-all is a useful medicinal plant used in many countries. Originating from Eurasia, it has now become naturalized in many countries. It is a low-sprawling perennial herb with small and purple or violet flowers.

Parts used:
stem, leaves, flowers: treat fever, tuberculosis of the lymphatic glands
fruits: treat headache, inflammation of the eyes, dizziness, anxiety, tuberculosis of the lymphatic glands

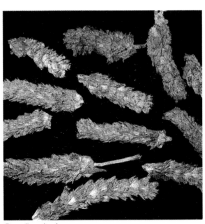

Prunella vulgaris

145

PRUNUS
FAMILY: Rosaceae
Prunus

The generic name for this group of plants, *Prunus*, is Latin for "plum". They are shrubs and trees mainly of northern temperate regions. Many are ornaments as well as stone fruits such as plums, almonds, apricots, peaches and cherries.

Prunus armeniaca 杏
common apricot

The common apricot is commonly planted for the fruits in the temperate areas of the northern hemisphere. The plant is native to China where it has been in cultivation since about 2000 B.C. The deciduous tree is rather attractive with its round crown and reddish bark. The leaves have toothed edges and are hairy along the veins on the lower surface. The solitary, pinkish or nearly white flowers appear before the emergence of new leaves, and develop into yellow or pale red, globular, velvety fruits. The flesh of the fruit is firm and sweet. However, excessive eating of the kernel can result in hydrocyanic acid poisoning.

The dried, ripe kernel is used medicinally throughout the East. It is considered a tonic and a purgative, with the ability to control spasms and expel phlegm from the respiratory passages. Seeds have been used against tumours in Europe as far back as A.D. 502. Apricot oil was also used for the same purpose in England during the 17th century. In more modern times laetrile, obtained from apricot pits and containing the substance, benzaldehyde, is used by Mexican physicians for the treatment of cancer. It is believed that once inside the body laetrile breaks down into several compounds including cyanide which acts on the tumour but not the healthy cells. This therapy is highly controversial and is illegal in the United States, Canada and many other countries. Japanese scientists are currently reexamining laetrile as a possible cancer cure.

Parts used:
kernel: treats common cold, coughs, bronchial asthma, rheumatism, constipation in old people
seeds: pain killer

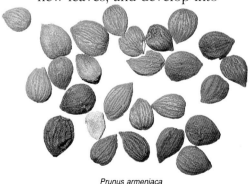
Prunus armeniaca

Prunus mume 梅
Japanese apricot
Japanese flowering apricot

The tree is taller than the common apricot, reaching 10 m, and just as attractive. It is native to China and southwestern Japan. In Japan it is a popular garden ornament and bonsai subject. Leaves are toothed along the edge and hairy along the veins on the undersurface. Flowers are in ones and twos, and white to dark red in colour. Fruits are round, yellow to greenish and slightly hairy. The flesh is sour and bitter.

Parts used:
unripe fruits: control fever, spasms, vomiting; expel intestinal worms; treat coughs, dysentery, chronic diarrhoea, irregular blood pressure, roundworm infections
petals: treat sore throat, fever
roots, bark: treat jaundice

Prunus japonica 郁李
Japanese plum
Japanese bush cherry
flowering almond

This is a small shrub, native to the region between China and Korea. The plant is much planted in Japan as an ornament and for its edible fruits.

Parts used:
whole plant: mild purgative; increases flow of urine; treats rheumatism, fever, indigestion

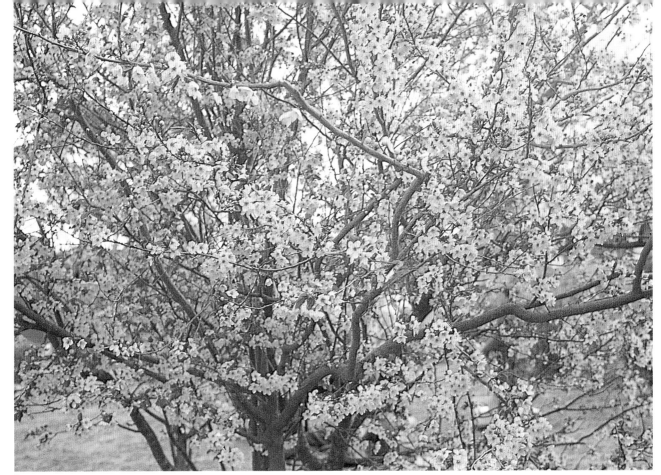

Prunus

Prunus persica 桃
peach

The peach is another attractive tree grown extensively in temperate countries for its fleshy fruits. It has leaves that are simple and large, and tooth-edged. The solitary, pink flowers appear after the fall of the leaves and well before the appearance of young leaves. Fruits are globular, with short hairs and yellow or red skin. The flesh is white or yellow, and there is a hard, pitted stone. The tree is native to China but it was once thought to come from Persia, hence the name *persica*. The kernel, flowers, leaves and bark contain hydrocyanic acid and can be poisonous. In ancient Egypt, condemned prisoners were caused to eat the ground kernels of the peach as a method of capital punishment, thus the phrase "penalty of the peach".

In many parts of the world peach leaves are used as a cure for whooping cough and the flowers (as well as the leaves) as a purgative and for the expelling of intestinal worms. Old English herbalists used powdered leaves and flowers to treat wounds; flowers in wine as a mild laxative; and a preparation of the leaves to treat inflammation of the stomach and bowels, as well as whooping cough. The bruised kernel, boiled in vinegar and applied to the bald head, was believed to cause hair to grow, where none grew before. In African folk medicine the leaves are given to girls whose menstruation is delayed.

Parts used:
kernel: induces menstruation; treats painful menstruation, internal bleeding, anaemia, appendicitis, constipation, coughs, rheumatism, bleeding of the uterus, hypertension
flowers: purgative; increase flow of urine

PSORALEA
FAMILY: Leguminosae
Psoralea corylifolia 补骨脂
scurfy pea

This shrub is native to Iran and India. It has characteristic black spots on the leaf surface. The yellow flowers are in prominent heads and borne on long stalks. They develop into one-seeded oval pods which, unlike most pods of the family, do not split open when ripe.

Parts used:
fruits, seeds: treat backache, aching bones resulting from the cold, irregular menstruation, yellow discharge from the vagina, excessive discharge of urine, involuntary discharge of urine, lumbago, diarrhoea
seeds: treat impotence, premature ejaculation

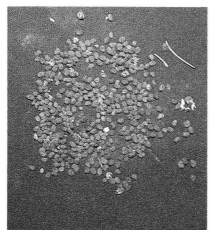

Psoralea corylifolia

PTERIDIUM
FAMILY: Polypodiaceae
Pteridium aquilinum 蕨
bracken

Bracken is also called "brake", meaning uncultivated land, in reference to its habitat, no doubt. The generic name, *Pteridium*, is from the Greek, *pteron*, or "wing", from the appearance of the leaves. The specific name *aquilinum* means "eagle-like". Many people consider the bracken a holy plant because when the stem is cut through, there is a broken circle pattern which is taken to represent Christ's monogram. The old English believed that growing the plant on the rooftop gave protection against lightning and thunder. Old English herbalists believed that plants collected during the waning of the moon was especially good for sprains and inflammation.

This fern is a northern hemisphere sun-loving, ground fern, thriving in well-drained soil and forming thickets. Its stem is underground, thus it is not easy to eradicate it once it establishes itself in any open areas. Setting fire to the plant only result in pure stands of the fern, as the parts above the ground, together with other plants, are burned off, allowing the underground stems to regenerate themselves.

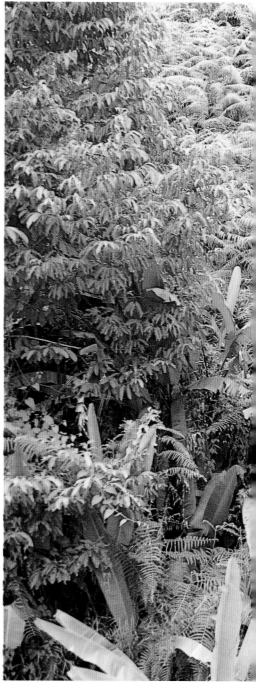

Pteridium aquilinum

148

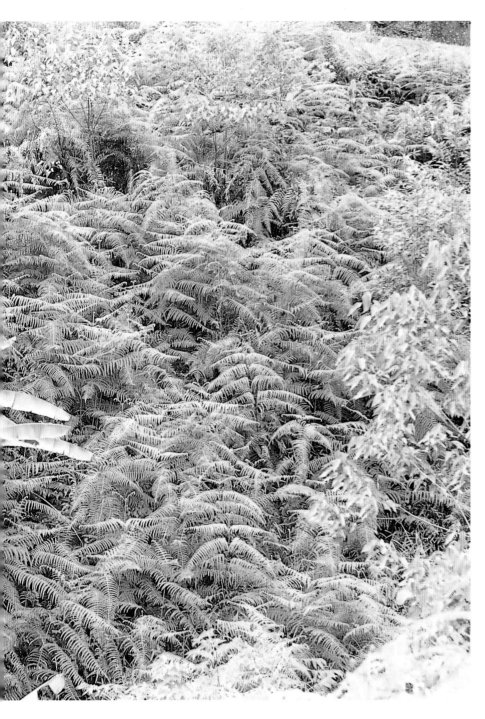

The starchy stem is eaten; young leaves are also eaten as a vegetable. The Japanese eat the young shoots as a green vegetable, as well as extract starch from the plant. Although the plant has been eaten, it has been known for a long time to poison livestock. However, it was only recently that the plant was discovered to have carcinogenic and mutigenic properties, and poisonous when consumed in large amounts. This can be one reason why there is a high incidence of stomach cancer among the Japanese.

Parts used:
stem: treats rheumatism.
stem, young shoots: purgative; cooling agents; increase the flow of urine; expel intestinal worms
leaf bases: treat rheumatism

PTERIS
FAMILY: Polypodiaceae
Pteris
brake

The generic name, *Pteris*, comes from the Greek word *pteron* meaning "wing", a general reference to ferns as they appear feathery or wing-like. The common name, brake, suggests the plant's habitat, as the word is derived from an Old English word meaning "uncultivated land". These ferns have their spore cases massed along the edge of the leaves in a continuous line.

Pteris multifida 凤尾草
spider brake
Chinese brake
This is a smallish fern of disturbed areas, native to East Asia but found in many tropical locations. The leaves are

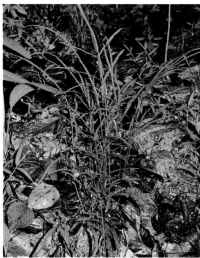

Pteris ensiformis

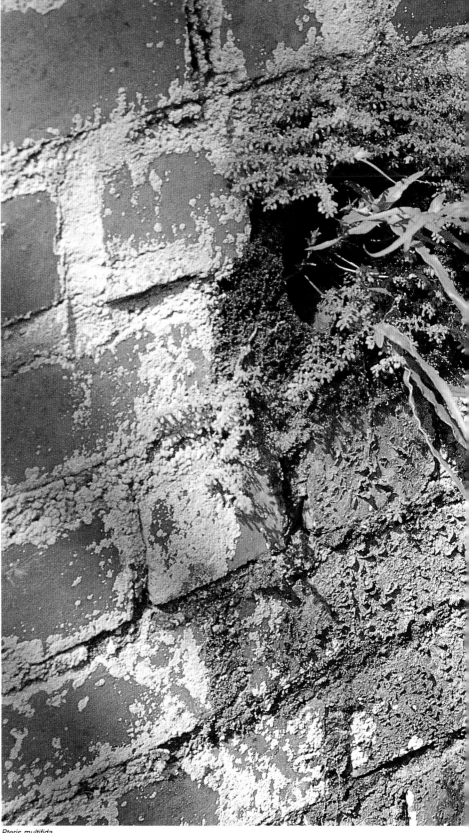

Pteris multifida

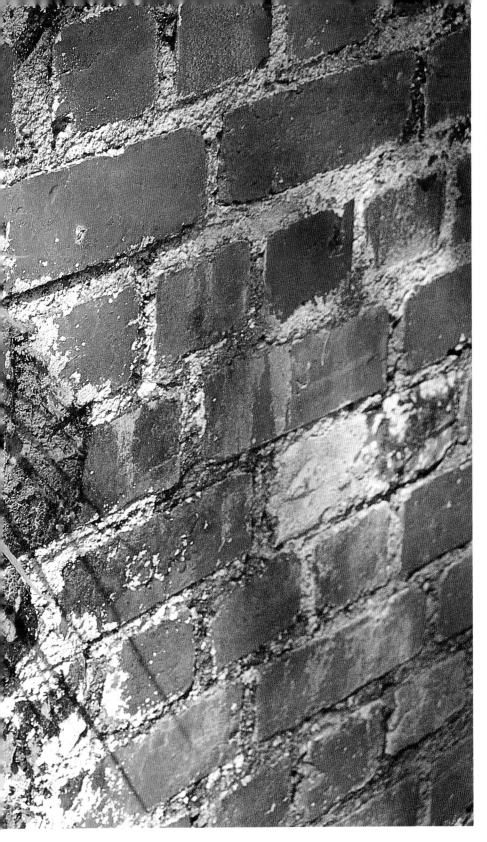

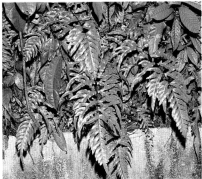

Pteris semipinnata

compound, consisting of two pairs of narrow leaflets and a terminal one, the lower pair of which is usually forked.

Parts used:
whole plant: purgative; expels intestinal worms; treats dysentery, jaundice, pain in the breast

Pteris ensiformis 劍叶凤尾草
This fern occurs commonly in open ground under shade.

Parts used:
whole plant: increases flow of urine; cools the system; wash for boils and piles; treats malaria, gonorrhoea, dysentery

Pteris actiniopteroides 半边旗
Parts used:
whole plant: promotes expulsion of phlegm from respiratory passages; stimulates gastric activities

Pteris semipinnata
Parts used:
whole plant: treats bites by poisonous snakes

151

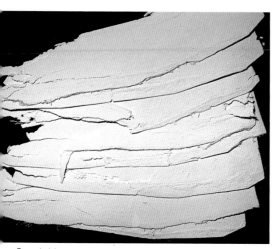

Pueraria lobata

PUERARIA
FAMILY: Leguminosae
Pueraria lobata 葛
kudzu vine

The plant is named after the European botanist, N. Pueraria (1765–1845). It is a woody, hairy vine, native to China and Japan. It is widely grown in southeastern United States for fodder, to control erosion and sometimes as an ornament. It is also cultivated in China and Japan for the textile fibres and for its roots, used in medicine. The usage of the plant in folk medicine is rather similar in China, Japan, Korea and Indochina.

Parts used:
roots: counter poisons; induce sweating; treat fever, vomiting, dysentery, diarrhoea, chicken pox, influenza, diabetes, typhoid fever, excessive gas in the system
flowers: treat excessive influence of alcoholic drinks, dysentery, gas in the intestine
vine (without the leaves): treats coughs, general weakness

PUNICA
FAMILY: Punicaceae
Punica granatum 石榴
pomegranate

Pomegranate comes from the Latin *pomum*, "apple", and *granatus*, "full of seeds". The botanical name comes from Old French, *pume grenate*, "pomegranate apple". Another interpretation has it that the botanical name is derived from an early name, *Malum punicum*, "apple of Carthage". The pomegranate is a very ancient plant, grown in the Hanging Gardens of Babylon. The origin of the plant is found in Greek mythology. A Scythian girl, told by some diviners that she was destined to one day wear the crown, bestowed her favours on Dionysus, god of productivity of nature, who promised to give her one. However, he soon became tired of her, whereupon she gradually pined away and died. Dionysus turned her into a pomegranate tree and placed a crown on the fruit (as represented by the calyx), to fulfill his promise.

The Chinese keep a pot of the plant handy in the garden or by the house, using a few leaves in water for bathing or to wash the face as a symbol of washing away bad luck or things evil. Because of the many seeds, it has also been regarded as a symbol of fertility by both Chinese and Greeks. The fruit skin has been used in tanning and as a fabric dye.

The pomegranate, native of the Mediterranean and West Asia, is now widely cultivated in tropical and subtropical countries for its edible fruit and as an ornament. It grows to a height of about 6 m. However, it takes to dwarfing, thus it is a favourite among bonsai enthusiasts. Branches are spiny, bearing smallish, narrow,

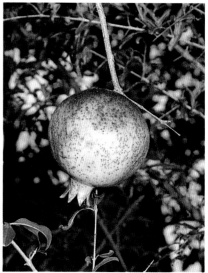

Punica granatum

oblong leaves. Flowers are solitary or in small clusters, large, orange-red, and rather showy. Fruits are rounded structures, ripening yellow to purplish-red. The thick skin encloses numerous, tightly-packed, wedge-shaped, edible, red-purple, juicy seeds.

Parts used:
fruit skin: treats diarrhoea, rectocele; expels pinworms
bark: treats piles, yellowish discharge from the vagina, sore throat, bad breath, nose bleed
leaves: relieve itch
flowers: treat burns

PYROLA
FAMILY: Pyrolaceae
Pyrola rotundifolia 鹿蹄草
wild lily-of-the-valley
wintergreen

The generic name is from the Greek *pyrus*, or "pear", as the foliage was thought to resemble the fruit. The plant has nearly round, thick, glossy leaves and white, fragrant flowers that are spirally arranged along an elongated stalk. It is native to Eurasia, Greenland, Newfoundland, East Quebec and Nova Scotia. The entire plant is used in Chinese medicine. It is collected with the roots, washed, dried under the sun until the leaves wrinkle, then piled and left to ferment.

The plants are then spread out in the sun and thoroughly dried. The best quality products are those with purplish leaves, a sign that they have been fermented; greyish leaves mean a substandard produce, as fermentation has not taken place.

Parts used:
whole plant: treats rheumatic pains, tuberculosis, general weakness, nervousness, blood in the sputum

PYRROSIA
FAMILY: Polypodiaceae
Pyrrosia lingua 石韦
tongue fern
Japanese felt fern

The generic name, *Pyrrosia* is derived from the Greek *pyrrhos*, meaning "fire-colour", in allusion to the colour of the spore sacs. This is a creeping fern found on trunks and branches of trees. The creeping stem is thin and wiry, and covered with scales, with leaves which are simple, lance-shaped and covered with a layer of brown hairs on the undersurface. The plant is native to China and Japan. Recent research has shown that it has properties that induce insects to shed their cuticle, as well as sedative and anti-spasmodic effects in animals.

Parts used:
whole plant: treats gonorrhoea, urinary difficulties such as painful discharge of urine, unusually plentiful or too little urine

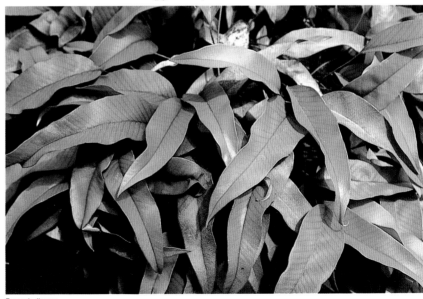

Pyrrosia lingua

153

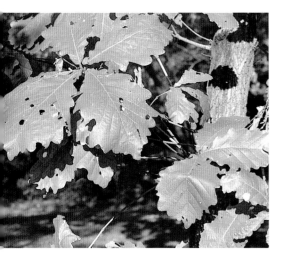

Quercus dentata

QUERCUS
FAMILY: Fagaceae
Quercus dentata 槲树
daimyo oak

The generic name, *Quercus*, is Latin for "tree". Oak trees were sacred to the sky and thunder gods, particularly Jupiter, the supreme deity of Roman mythology. For this reason it was known as the tree of Jove and it was believed that lightning would not strike an oak tree in a storm. The daimyo oak is native to Korea, Japan and China.

Parts used:
acorns: treat diarrhoea, excessive bleeding during menstruation
leaves: quench thirst; stop bleeding; treat piles, dysentery
bark: expels intestinal worms

QUISQUALIS
FAMILY: Combretaceae
Quisqualis indica 使君子
Rangoon creeper

Quisqualis in Latin means "What is this?" and refers to the changing colour of the flower from white through pink to red, as well as the arrangement of the leaves along the stem, which varies from alternate to opposite pairs to threes. The plant is a fast-growing climbing shrub, capable of growing to a height of 10 m. The lower portion of the leaf stalk remains on the stem after the leaf has fallen, to become hard and thorn-like. Flowers are in terminal drooping bunches, fragrant, and white turning pink or red. The plant is native to Burma, Peninsular Malaysia, the Philippines and New Guinea. Extracts of the plant have been shown experimentally to possess antitumour properties when tested on animals.

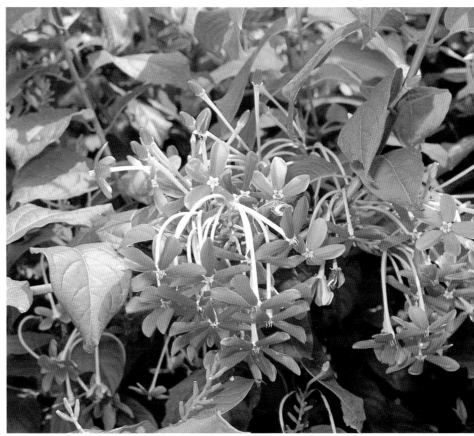

Quisqualis indica

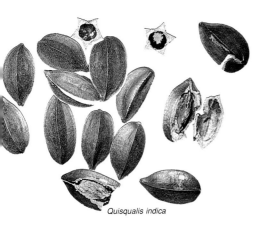

Quisqualis indica

Parts used:
fruits, seeds: treat roundworm infestation, swelling of the belly
seeds in oil: treat skin diseases, boils and sores on faces of children

RAPHANUS
FAMILY: Cruciferae
Raphanus sativus 莱菔
radish

This is planted for its fleshy roots which are eaten as a vegetable. Leaves are much dissected while the white or purplish flowers are small and in loose bunches. The radish has been used in the traditional medicines of Japan, Indochina and India.

Parts used:
roots: aid digestion
seeds: expel phlegm from

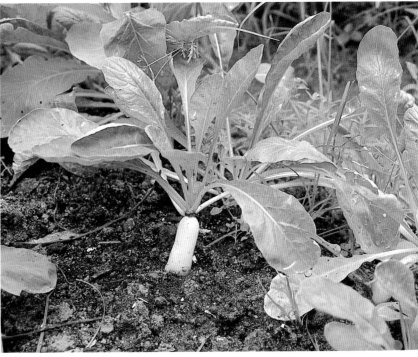

Raphanus sativus

respiratory passages
leaves: treat headache
whole plant: treats diarrhoea, dysentery, malnutrition, coughs; expels intestinal worms

REHMANNIA
FAMILY: Scrophulariaceae
Rehmannia glutinosa 地黄
rehmannia

Rehmannia is named after the physician from Leningrad, Joseph Rehmann (1779–1831). It is a perennial herb, native to northern China. The purple, hairy plant has a basal rosette of leaves, from which arise the

erect flowering stem. The flowers are dull, purple-brown or creamy-white, and densely covered with glandular hairs. Fresh or dried roots have been used medicinally in China since time immemorial. The roots, yellowish and tasting sweetish, are dried over a slow fire.

Parts used:
roots: cooling agent; purgative; stop bleeding; treat fever, vomiting of blood, ulcers in the mouth, anaemia, weak liver or kidney, lumbago, sore throat, irregular menstruation, premature ejaculation, dizziness

155

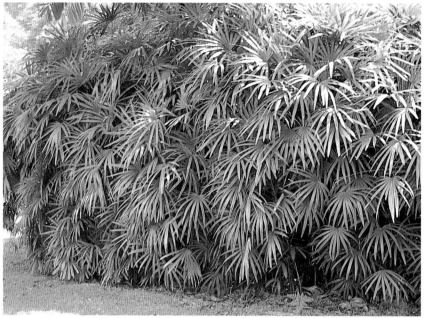
Rhapis excelsa

RHAPIS
FAMILY: Palmae
Rhapis excelsa 棕竹
lady palm
bamboo palm
slender lady palm
miniature fan-palm
China cane
partridge cane

This palm is well known as a pot plant. It originated from southern China but is now found throughout the world as an ornamental palm. It grows in clumps of four palms. The leaves, spaced along the length of the stem, are split palmately into five to ten or more segments.

Parts used:
leaf stalk, bark, fruits: stop bleeding
root: stimulates blood circulation; treats rheumatism

RHEUM
FAMILY: Polygonaceae
Rheum tanguticum 唐古特大黄
rhubarb

The generic name comes from *rha*, the old Greek word for rhubarb. These plants are native to Asia and well known for their purgative action, due to the presence of anthraquinones. In low dosage the plant has purgative action, while in high dosage it checks diarrhoea because of the predominant action of the tannin contents.

Parts used:
roots: treat intestinal or stomach fever, constipation, acute infectious hepatitis, jaundice, diarrhoea, absence of menstruation due to blood clot, internal bleeding

RHIZOPHORA
FAMILY: Rhizophoraceae
Rhizophora mucronata 红茄苳
bakau kurap

This is a typical tree of the tropics, with prominent stilt roots growing out from the trunks in an effort to stabilize the plant in a swampy habitat. Thus a grove of *bakau* trees would be closely intertwined by the numerous stilt roots developing from all directions. *Bakau kurap* is one of the most common mangrove trees of this region. The poles of this tree are in demand for piling and for the construction of houses bordering these swamps. The wood is also valued for firewood and for the making of charcoal. The bark was once used to tan leather.

Parts used:
bark: treats diarrhoea

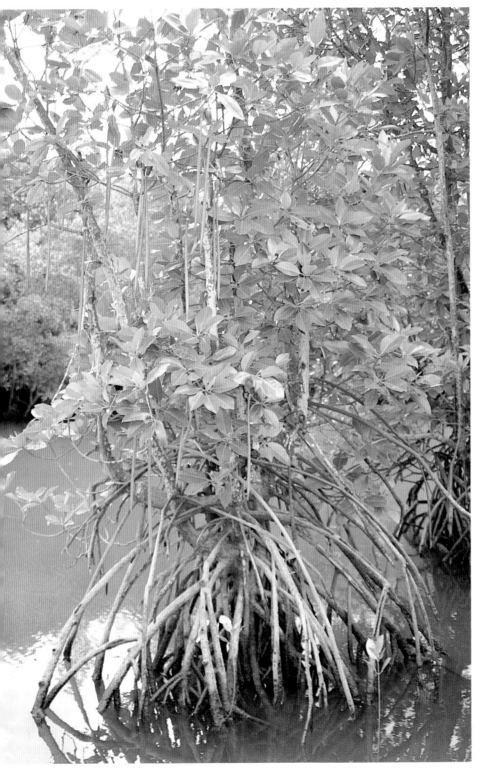

ora mucronata

RHOEO
FAMILY: Commelinaceae
Rhoeo spathacea 紫万年青
purple-leaved spider wort
boat lily
Moses-in-the-cradle
two-men-in-a-boat

This is an attractive foliage plant native to the West Indies, Mexico and Guatemala. The plant has long, narrow, pointed leaves which are dark green on the upper and purple on the lower surface. Flowers are small and white, and concealed within a boat-shaped envelope of two bracts.

Parts used:
flowers: treat intestinal bleeding, blood in the sputum, dysentery

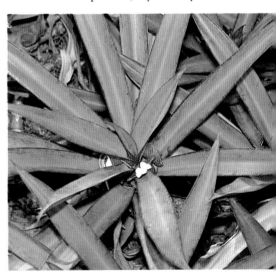

Rhoeo spathacea

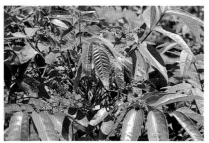
Rhus verniciflua

RHUS
FAMILY: Anacardiaceae
Rhus
sumach

Sumach are any temperate or subtropical small trees or shrubs of the genus *Rhus*, which is an ancient Greek name. Many of these plants are grown as ornaments, for the colourful autumn foliage or the colourful fruits. The dried leaves of a number of species yield tannin, while others produce lacquers. The sap of some are poisonous, causing dermatitis on contact.

Rhus verniciflua 漆树
Japanese lacquer tree
varnish tree
This species is native to temperate East Asia. It is cultivated in southwestern Japan as a source of lacquer. The fresh sap causes dermatitis on contact but hardened sap is quite harmless.

Parts used:
hardened sap: increases menstrual flow; expels intestinal worms

Rhus succedanea 木蜡树
wax tree
The wax tree is cultivated for its berries, which are a source of a commercial wax, used in the production of ointments. The stamens give off a substance which is used as natural lacquer.

Parts used:
fruit wax: used in ointments

Rhus javanica 盐肤木
nutgall tree
Rhus potanini 青麸杨
Rhus punjabensis var. *sinica* 红麸杨
Parts used:
galls developing from the midrib of the leaflet, axis of leaf: treat sores, diarrhoea, bleeding, dysentery, tuberculosis

RICINUS
FAMILY: Euphorbiaceae
Ricinus communis 蓖麻
castor-oil plant
castor-bean
palma christi

The plant is native to the tropics, but now naturalized in almost every region of the world, and commonly grown as an ornament. The flowers are without petals, the males and females in the same dense, terminal bunches which are often 30 to 60 cm long. Normally, the upper clusters of flowers are males while the lower clusters females. Fruits are three-lobed, roundish and spiny, and borne on a long stalk. They are green, turning brown on ripening, when they split open to expose three smooth, marbled seeds.

The seeds yield an oil which the ancient Egyptians used as an illuminant. In the West, castor oil was mainly used as a purgative, up to the early 20th century. Now the oil is used in industry, to coat fabrics; in the manufacture of high grade lubricants, soaps, paints, varnishes and printing ink; in textile dyeing; for the preservation of leather; and in the cosmetic industry. The seeds are poisonous, containing a toxic protein, ricin, which acts as a blood coagulant. A single seed, if not fatal, may cause serious illness. The poison acts slowly, the first symptom appearing about 10 hours after ingestion, which is vomiting. This is followed by diarrhoea, cold sweat, a burning sensation in the mouth, thirst, the skin turning blue, heart disorder, convulsions, and, finally, death from respiratory failure and cardiac arrest.

Parts used:
seeds: treat abscesses and skin eruptions, deafness, headache, skin problems, bleeding, constipation, boils, piles; promote labour

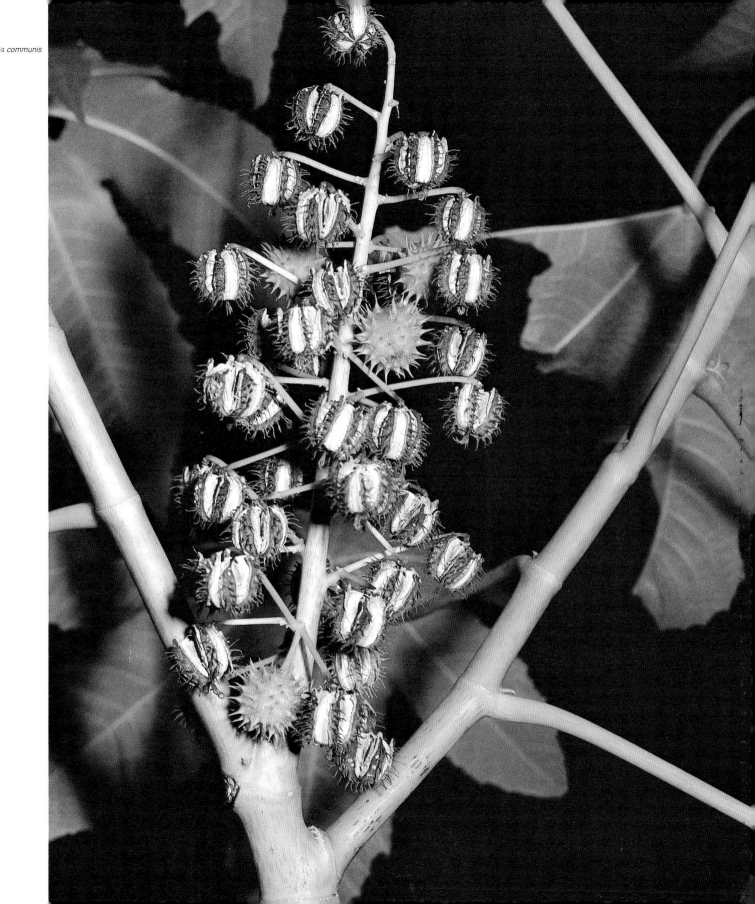

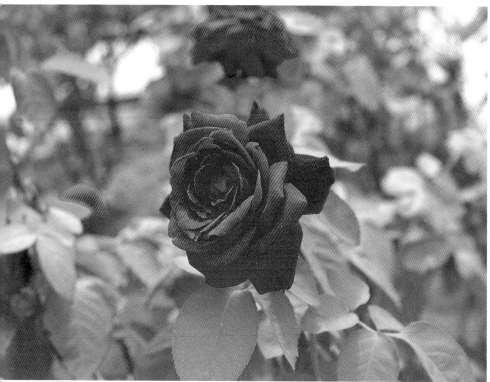

Rosa

ROSA
FAMILY: Rosaceae
Rosa
rose

Roses are northern temperate shrubs or scrambling plants, and typically prickly. The origin of the generic name, *Rosa*, may have come from the Celtic *rhos* or the Greek *rodon*, both meaning "red". The flower is a symbol of the western world and became the national flower of England during the War of the Roses (1455–85). In Greek mythology Venus presented the rose to her son Cupid, who in turn gave it to Harpocrates, the god of silence, to induce him to conceal the weaknesses of the gods. Thus the rose came to represent silence. In certain European countries it was customary to hang a rose from the ceiling when secrecy was required. The plants are grown for their ornamental value or for the essential oils, obtained from certain species, and used in the production of perfumes.

Rosa laevigata 金櫻子
Cherokee rose
This rose is native to China. It is an evergreen scrambler covered with hooked spines and has fragrant, white flowers. It is believed that the high tannin content of the plant is responsible for its effectiveness against diarrhoea.

Parts used:
fruits: treat premature ejaculation, yellowish discharge from the vagina, incontinence, inflammation of uterus and intestine, diarrhoea

Rosa chinensis 月季花
Chinese rose
Parts used:
petals: treat irregular menstruation, pain in the lower portion of the stomach

RUBIA
FAMILY: Rubiaceae
Rubia cordifolia 茜草
Indian madder

The Indian madder is a creeping weed from China, India and Africa. The stem, squarish in cross-section, bears heart-shaped leaves on long stalks; leaves have prickles along the edge. Flowers are in terminal bunches, small and yellow-white. The generic name *Rubia* comes from the Latin word *ruber*, meaning "red", a reference to the colour of a dye extracted from the roots.

Parts used:
roots: tonic for the blood system; treat excessive or an absence of menstruation, blood in vomit or sputum, blood in urine, rheumatoid arthritis, jaundice, dysentery

RUBUS
FAMILY: Rosaceae
Rubus parvifolius 茅莓
Japanese bramble

Brambles are found all over the world, but are mainly distributed in the northern hemisphere. These include blackberries, dewberries and raspberries, sought after for the fruits, which are either harvested from the wild or cultivated. The generic name *Rubus* comes from the Latin word *ruber* meaning "red". In the Christian tradition the European bramble is an emblem of Christ and the Virgin Mary. It is also a Hebrew symbol of divine love and the voice of God.

This prickly plant grows in wastelands, bearing reddish fruits, which consist of a number of fruitlets in a bunch. The dried fruits are rough, roundish structures, which are light brown in colour.

Parts used:
roots, leaves: treat skin problems
unripe fruits: tonic; aphrodisiac

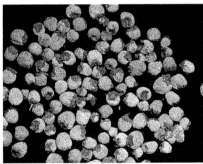
Rubus parvifolius

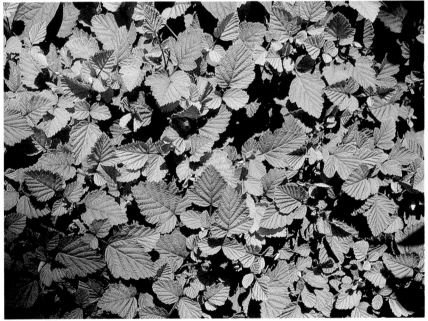
Rubus parvifolius

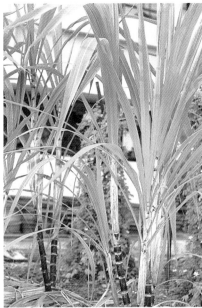
Saccharum officinarum

SACCHARUM
FAMILY: Gramineae
Saccharum officinarum 甘蔗
sugar cane

Saccharum is an old Greek term for sugar. The plant is grown for the sugar it contains; cane sugar provides more than half the world's supply of sugar. The plant is native to the Old World tropics, introduced into America by Columbus. One of the reasons for the development of the slave trade in the United States was the high labour requirement of this crop. It is now planted in the tropics as well as the subtropics.

Parts used:
cane juice: promotes expulsion of phlegm from the respiratory passages; stimulates gastric activities; treats wounds, ulcers, boils

SALIX
FAMILY: Salicaceae
Salix
willow

Willows are native mainly to the colder and temperate regions of the northern hemisphere. Many are ornaments, or grown for shelter, screen and erosion control. The generic name comes from the Celtic *salis*, meaning "near water". Willows have a long history in medicinal usage. The Greeks of old made use of the bark from various willows as a pain reliever and to treat gout and other illnesses.

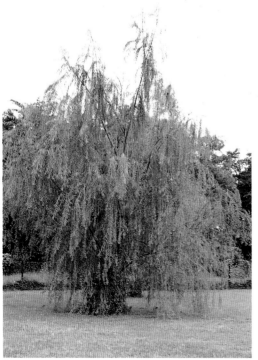
Salix babylonica

Similarly, the North American Indians used the bark of the plant to contain fever, relieve the aches and pains of rheumatism, and treat lumbago and headache. However, it was only in the 19th century that the glucoside salicin, an effective pain killer, was isolated from these plants. For a long time salicin was actually used for this purpose until it was replaced by synthetic drugs like aspirin. The main commercial source of salicin, used for rheumatism, are brittle willow (*Salix fragilis*) and basket willow (*Salix purpurea*).

Salix babylonica 垂柳
weeping willow
This is a medium-sized tree, native probably to China, and popularly planted in parks and gardens. The Swedish botanist, Linnaeus, who was the first to describe the plant, thought it came from the Babylonian region, thus the specific name, *babylonica*. The branches are long-hanging, giving the tree a weeping appearance, thus the common name, weeping willow.

Parts used:
young shoots: treat abscesses, ulcers, skin diseases, measles
twigs: treat rheumatism, gonorrhoea
gum: treat sores
shoot/root bark: treat jaundice, rheumatism, fever, gonorrhoea

Salix pentandra
bay willow
bay-leaved willow
laurel willow
This plant is of European origin but cultivated in China.

Parts used:
bark: treats abscesses

Salix purpurea 红皮柳
basket willow
Parts used:
bark: treats rheumatism
twigs, leaves: treat chronic dysentery, smallpox ulcers

SALVIA
FAMILY: Labiatae
Salvia
sage

The generic name, *Salvia*, comes fron the Latin *salveo*, "I heal", in reference to the reputed properties of the plant. These are herbs and shrubs found widely throughout the world, on dry and stony areas. The common sage was thought to soothe grief, and its leaves were strewn on graves for remembrance as they wilt very slowly. In certain cases the plant was grown on graves. The leaves were used by young maidens in old England as oracles, mainly to get a glimpse of their future husbands.

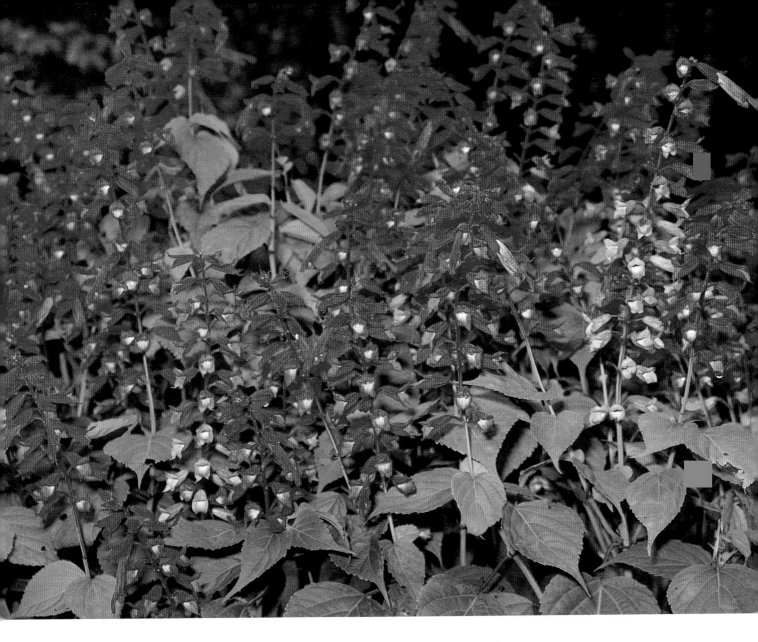

Salvia miltiorrhiza 丹參
Chinese sage
The plant comes from northeastern China, Manchuria and Japan. The dry roots, which are medicinal, are available as forked, slender pieces, brick red, wrinkled and brittle. Because of the redness, they are used in problems related with blood.

Parts used:
roots: treat absence of and painful menstruation, bleeding in the uterus, inflammation of the breast, bone and kidneys, pain in the stomach, ulcers of the liver, stomach and large intestine, internal abscesses, heart palpitation, insomnia

Salvia japonica
Japanese sage
Parts used:
leaves, flowers: treat enlarged organs, parasitic worms, malarial fever, dropsy

SANGUISORBA
FAMILY: Rosaceae
Sanguisorba officinalis 地榆
burnet
burnet bloodwort

Burnets are herbs from the northern temperate zones. The generic name comes from the Latin, *sanguis*, "blood", and *sorbes*, "to absorb", meaning "blood-stopping", in reference to the reputed medicinal properties of the plant. The roots of the burnet are collected, sliced, and roasted until they are black. The fresh roots are red and thus used to treat problems related to blood.

Parts used:
roots: treat excessive bleeding after labour, excessive bleeding during menstruation, coughing of blood, burns, inflammation of the skin, diarrhoea, dysentery

SCHISANDRA
FAMILY: Schisandraceae
Schisandra chinensis 北五味子
magnolia vine

A twining shrub from temperate East Asia, the magnolia vine is frequently planted for the decorative red berries. The dried ripe berries have been used medicinally in China for more than 2000 years.

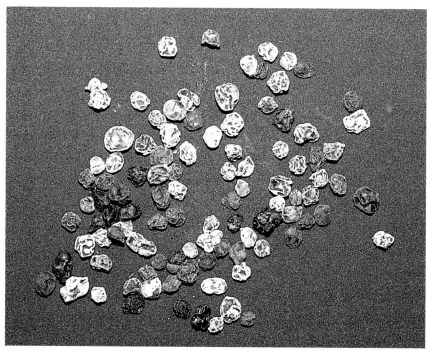
Schisandra chinensis

Parts used:
fruits: tonic; cool the body system; improve digestion, blood circulation; treat coughs, asthma, premature ejaculation, sweating during the night, dysentery, insomnia

SCROPHULARIA
FAMILY: Scrophulariaceae
Scrophularia
figwort

The generic name is derived from the disease called scrofula, commonly known as King's Evil because the monarch's hand is supposed to have miraculous powers to cure it. The plant is a strong-scented herb, native to the northern hemisphere. The stem is four-angled, from which arise leaves in opposite pairs. Flowers are small and non-showy, and green, purple, red or yellow.

Scrophularia buergeriana 北玄參
A native of northern China, Korea, Manchuria and Japan, the plant usually grows in grassy areas along rivers in the lowlands. This herb has a swollen, fleshy rootstock which bears erect four-angled stems.

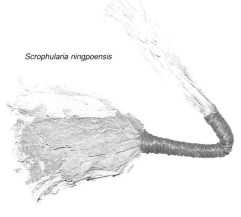

Scrophularia ningpoensis

Parts used:
roots: tonic for the heart; treat fever, malaria, kidney disease, typhoid fever, yellowish discharge from the vagina

Scrophularia ningpoensis 玄参
Parts used:
roots: treat fever, sore throat, anxiety, vomiting of blood, nose bleeds, rash, difficulty in urination, boils, constipation

SCUTELLARIA
FAMILY: Labiatae
Scutellaria baicalensis 黄芩
skullcap

The generic name means "dish" in Latin, and refers to the dish-like form of the persistent calyx of the flower. The plant is a spreading herb, native to East Asia. Unlike the other members of the family, these plants are bitter and not aromatic.

Parts used:
roots: treat high fever, dry coughs, vomiting of blood, constipation, hypertension, inflammation of the breast, jaundice, diarrhoea; prevent spontaneous abortion

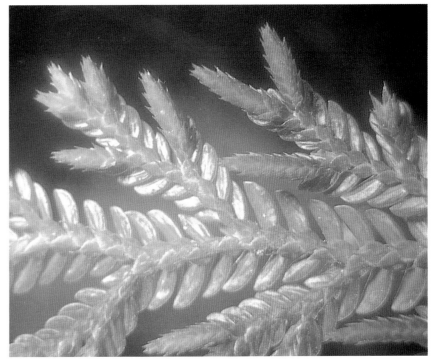

Selaginella

SELAGINELLA
FAMILY: Labiatae
Selaginella involvens 兖卷柏
spikemoss

This herbaceous plant has two types of leaves – a pair of larger outer rows, and an inner pair of smaller rows. Under dry conditions the plant curls up, but when there is moisture, it revives. Because of this behaviour of "dying and yet not dying", the plant is thought to have the capability to prolong life. It is thus used by the Chinese in problems related to the aged.

Parts used:
whole plant: tonic for internal injuries; enhances menstrual flow; expels intestinal worms; treats coughs, including coughing of blood, old age problems

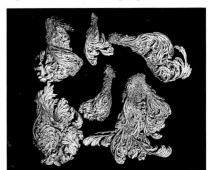

Selaginella involvens

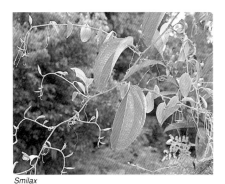
Smilax

SMILAX
Family: Liliaceae
Smilax glabra 土茯苓
greenbrier

Greenbrier is a woody vine with an enlarged underground stem. The roots of several tropical American species yield sarsaparilla, used medicinally, and as a flavouring. The plant is also used as an insecticide.

Parts used:
whole plant: cooling tonic; purgative; treats boils, abscesses

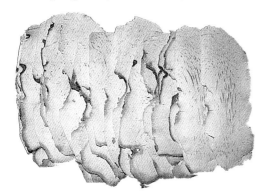
Smilax glabra

SOLANUM
FAMILY: Solanaceae
Solanum nigrum 龙葵
common nightshade
black nightshade
poisonberry

The plant comes from Europe but is now widely distributed. The generic name, *Solanum*, is said to be from the Latin, *solamen*, "quieting", an allusion to the sedative qualities of the plant. It is a herb which bears black berries containing many kidney-shaped seeds. The unripe fruits and leaves are said to be poisonous due to the presence of steroidal alkaloids. The controversial nature of its toxicity can be due to the variation in toxic chemical contents in relation to location, time of the year and other factors. Again, there may be confusion in plant identification in the different reports of poisoning. However, the leaves are consumed in some countries as a vegetable and the berries made into pies and preserves.

The Europeans in Africa use the plant to treat convulsions while the Africans themselves use it for headache, ulcers, wounds and as a sedative. It would appear that the plant has a common usage in a number of cultures as a sedative, since ancient times.

Parts used:
whole plant: treats dermatitis, inflammation, heavy female discharge, sore throat, diarrhoea, dysentery

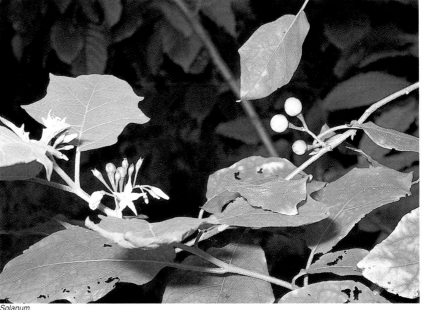
Solanum

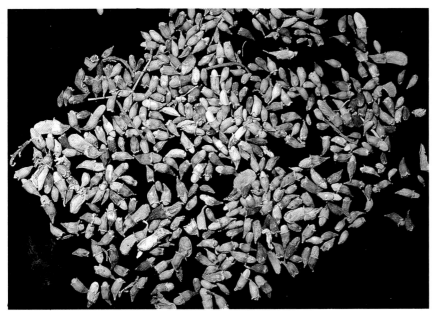
Sophera japonica

SOPHERA
FAMILY: Leguminosae
Sophera
sophera

Sophera is an Arabic term for the tree, which bears pea-shaped flowers. This woody plant, of wide distribution, has cylindrical or four-angled fruits which are constricted between seeds. Many are showy in blossoms and are thus popular ornaments.

Sophera japonica 槐
Chinese scholar tree
Japanese pagoda tree
This tree is native to China, Korea and northern Vietnam. It has a round-headed crown and white to yellow flowers, which develop into hairy, cylindrical, fleshy pods. The flower buds give a colouring matter which is an important commercial source of quercetin. They are also used in the brewing of beer.

Parts used:
flower buds, fruits, seeds: arrest bleeding; treat coughing of blood, blood in the faeces, menstrual clots, hypertension, piles
fruit: expels intestinal worms

Sophera flavescens 苦参
This shrub is native to China, and has been used as an insecticide.

Parts used:
roots: treat diarrhoea, piles, jaundice, swollen ankles, fever, sore throat, intestinal bleeding, syphilis, leprosy, toothache, asthma

Sophera subprostrata 广豆根
In powder form the roots are used to treat snake bites and boils. The plant has been shown to have antitumour substances.

Parts used:
seeds: cool the body system; treat sore throat, cough, laryngitis, constipation, gum inflammation, acute bile duct inflammation, jaundice

SPARGANIUM
FAMILY: Sparganiaceae
Sparganium stoloniferum 黑三棱
sparganium

The herb thrives in wet habitats in northern temperate regions. The grasslike leaves are long and narrow and flowers are small and gathered in heads.

Parts used:
underground stem: treats internal bleeding; increases menstrual flow; induces abortion; induces secretion of milk in women after labour; sedative

STEMONA
FAMILY: Stemonaceae

Stemona sessilifolia 直立百部
stemona

Stemona comes from East and Southeast Asia, northern Australia, and the southeastern part of the United States. It is a herb, with large, greenish, bell-shaped flowers. Tubers are collected just after the old shoot dies or after the emergence of the new shoot. They are used untreated, or dipped in boiling water and dried before use. Sometimes they are treated in honey after being dipped in boiling water.

Parts used:
tubers: remove lice from the head; treat tuberculosis, coughs, whooping cough, sore throat, skin diseases

TETRAPANAX
FAMILY: Araliaceae

Tetrapanax papyriferus 通脱木
Chinese rice-paper plant
rice-paper plant

Native to southern China and Taiwan, the small tree is planted for the white stem pith, used to make rice paper. Shoots are covered with a white layer of felt-like hairs, which becomes rusty in colour with age. The large, deeply lobed leaves are similarly densely hairy on the underside. Flowers are

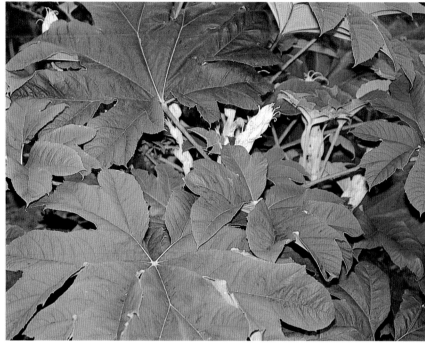

Tetrapanax papyriferus

yellowish-white, and arranged in small globular bunches, which in turn make up one large bunch. This is borne on a 1 m tall stalk, the whole standing out prominently beyond the leaves.

The sweetish stem pith is used medicinally. It is believed to have cooling effects, and has shown to possess anticancer properties when tested on laboratory animals. Year-old suckers are cut into short lengths and the pith pushed out with the aid of a stick.

Parts used:
stem pith: treats coughs, fever, diabetes; induces the flow of milk in women after labour; induces flow of urine; expels intestinal worms

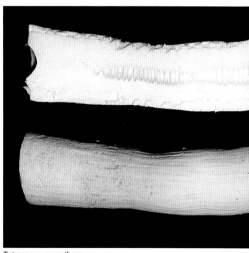

Tetrapanax papyriferus

168

TORREYA
FAMILY: Taxaceae
Torreya nucifera 榧
kaya
Japanese torreya
stinking yew

This is an evergreen tree with reddish brown branches, native to Japan. The seeds, looking like acorns, are about 2 cm long and have an outer green covering which is tinged with purple. They are edible and are rich in oil.

Parts used:
seeds: laxative; expel intestinal worms

TRACHELOSPERMUM
FAMILY: Apocynaceae
Trachelospermum jasminoides 络石
star jasmine
confederate jasmine

This is an evergreen woody vine of 10 m or more in length, sometimes grown as an ornament because of its fragrant flowers. It is native to southern China. The generic name, *Trachelospermum*, comes from the Greek words *trachelos* and *sperma* for "neck" and "seed" respectively.

Parts used:
stem, leaves: tonic; pain killer; increase menstrual flow; treat sore throat, arthritis, rheumatism

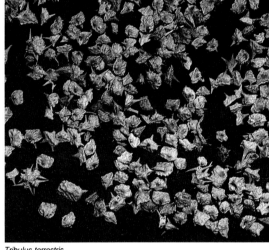
Tribulus terrestris

TRIBULUS
FAMILY: Zygophyllaceae
Tribulus terrestris 蒺藜
burnut
puncture vine

This is a low herb, native to the Old World tropics, but now naturalized in many tropical countries. The hard fruit splits into three when ripe; each part has four spines and the entire structure appears star-shaped.

Parts used:
fruits: tonic; aphrodisiac; induce abortion; improve appetite; increase menstrual flow; induce milk secretion in women after labour; expel intestinal worms; stop bleeding; relieve headache; treat dizziness, chest congestion, eye inflammation, premature ejaculation, nervous breakdown

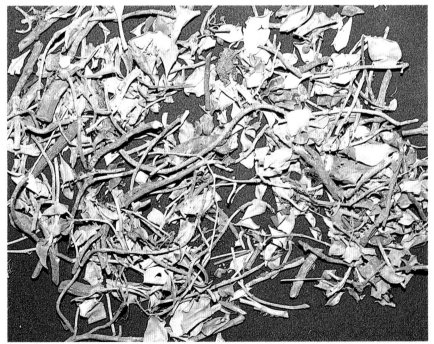
Trachelospermum jasminoides

TRICHOSANTHES
FAMILY: Cucurbitaceae

Trichosanthes kirilowii 栝楼
trichosanthes

The generic name, *Trichosanthes*, is Greek, meaning "hair-flower", and refers to the fringed petals. The plant is a vine of southern China and Vietnam. The stem bears many three- to five-branched tendrils and three-lobed leaves. Roots are fleshy, and taste bittersweet. Fruits are rounded and fleshy, and used in dried form medicinally, together with the seeds. The roots are dug out in autumn, bleached in sulphur fumes, and dried.

Parts used:
roots: treat constipation, fever, chest congestion, anxiety, inflammation of the breast, diabetes
starch from the fleshy roots: treat ulcers, chicken pox, skin diseases

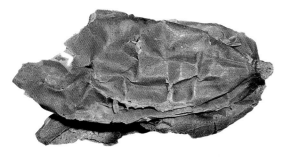
Trichosanthes kirilowii

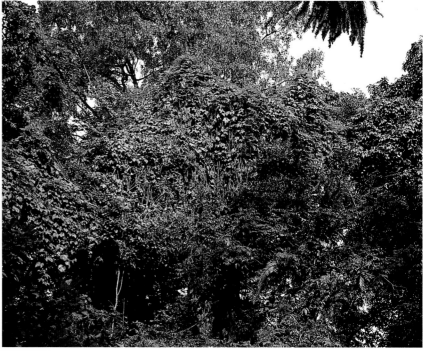
Trichosanthes

TUSSILAGO
FAMILY: Compositae

Tussilago farfara 款冬
coltsfoot

Coltsfoot is so named because the shape of the leaves resembles the foot of the colt. Other common names are ass's-foot, horsehoof, hallfoot and bullsfoot. The generic name, *Tussilago*, comes from the Latin, *tussis* and *agere*, "to take away the cough", as the plant was used to treat coughs. The English used to tell the weather by observing the fruiting heads of the plant in summer. If the hairs were blown off when there was no wind, there was impending rain. Old European herbalists used the plant to treat chest complaint. Pliny, the Roman author of the celebrated *Natural History* suggested that the dried leaves and roots be burnt over cypress charcoal and the smoke drawn into the mouth and swallowed as a remedy for cough. The plant was mixed with yarrow and rose leaves and used as a herbal tobacco to cure asthma.

This herbaceous plant has large, heart-shaped leaves, borne on long stalks, rising from the base in a rosette. It originates from the Old World countries of Europe, western and northern Asia and North Africa. It has become naturalized in the eastern regions of North America. It has a licorice-like fragrance and is used in the curing of pipe tobacco. Fresh leaves are sometimes eaten as a vegetable while the dried leaves are made into a tea and drunk as an ancient Chinese remedy against coughs. Pectins have been isolated from the leaves of the plant. As these substances have soothing effects, this could account for the effectiveness of the leaves against coughs.

Parts used:
flower buds: treat coughs with blood, asthma, bronchitis, lung cancer

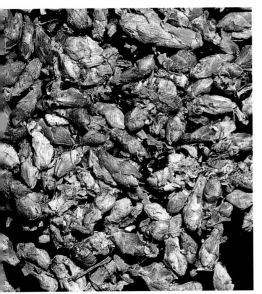
go farfara

TYPHA
FAMILY: Typhaceae
Typha
cattails
cattail flag
reed-mace
bulrush

The generic name, *Typha*, comes from the Greek *typhos*, meaning "marsh", and refers to the natural habitat of the plant. Bulrushes are tall plants of swamps and marshes, native to North America, Europe and Asia. The 2 m high plant has stiff, narrow leaves of up to 3 m long. The flowers are small, and borne in a dense, spike-like structure, thus the common name cattail. At maturity the spike appears brown to black. Plants are commonly grown in aquatic gardens. The dried leaves are used for matting while the dried fruiting spikes for floral arrangement. The downy tufts were used to stuff pillows and mattresses in England and the long leaves as thatching materials as well as for making mats and baskets.

Typha angustifolia	狭叶香蒲
Typha bungeana	香蒲
Typha davidiana	线叶香蒲
Typha minima	小香蒲
Typha orientalis	东方香蒲
Typha latifolia	宽叶香蒲

These are all found in China and used medicinally, the different species not being

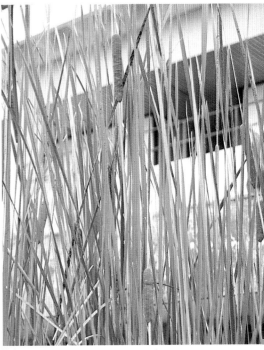
Typha

distinguished. The dried yellow pollen is collected and used uncooked as an anticoagulant or cooked as a coagulant. The pollen is sometimes roasted over a slow fire until black and used to stop bleeding.

Parts used:
pollen: treats blood in the urine, painful and absence of menstruation, urinary troubles, abdominal pain, vomiting of blood, internal bleeding
underground stem: tonic; increases flow of urine; induces secretion of milk in women after childbirth; treats dysentery; controls fever

171

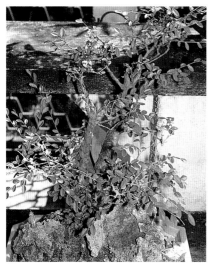
Ulmus

ULMUS
FAMILY: Ulmaceae
Ulmus pumila 榆树
dwarf elm
Siberian elm

The generic name of elm, *Ulmus*, is the Latin name of the tree. Elms are magnificent trees, favourite for shade and along avenues. They were once widespread in the northern temperate countries but the epidemic of Dutch elm disease of the 1920's killed off thousands of these trees and, even today, only a few areas are disease-free. The dwarf elm is a small tree, sometimes shrublike, with slender and drooping branches. It is native to eastern Siberia, northern and eastern China and Turkestan, and cultivated elsewhere.

Parts used:
leaves: increase flow of urine; reduce fever; remove stones from the bladder
inner bark: treats various skin eruptions, abscesses and swellings, diarrhoea, backache, sweating at night, ringing in the ear

UNCARIA
FAMILY: Rubiaceae
Uncaria
uncaria

The name *Uncaria* comes from the Latin *uncus*, meaning "hook", as these plants bear on their stems, strong, downward-curving hooks. They are all climbing shrubs of the forest with flowers in large, ball-shaped heads.

Uncaria rhynchophylla 钩藤
This species is native to China and Japan.

Parts used:
vine: treats children suffering from convulsions and other nervous disorders

Uncaria sinensis 华钩藤
Parts used:
vine: sedative; treats fever, headache, dizziness, nervous disorders, colds, convulsions

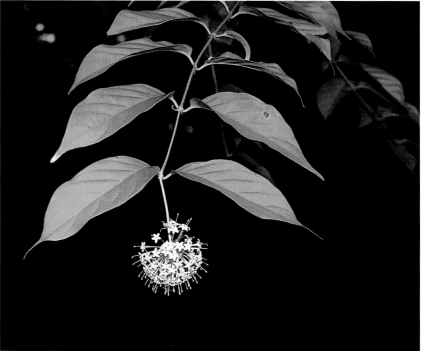
Uncaria

VACCARIA
FAMILY: Caryophyllaceae
Vaccaria pyramidata 麦蓝菜
cow herb
dairy pink

This herb is native to Europe and Asia. The plant was believed to be a good cattle fodder, hence the name *vacca*, Latin for "cow", and the common name, cow herb. The stem is erect and forked, and the flowers pink to dark purple.

Parts used:
seeds: treat inflammation of the breast, benign breast tumour, absence of lactation following labour; induce menstruation

VALERIANA
FAMILY: Valerianaceae
Valeriana officinalis 缬草
common valerian
drunken sailor

Valerian comes from the Latin *valere*, "to be healthy", on account of the medicinal virtues of the plant. Others attribute the name to Valerius, a physician who was said to be the first person to have used the plant medicinally. The plant, a native to West Asia and Europe, gives the official drug valerian. It has a strong and intoxicating odour, especially when bruised, from which no doubt comes the common English name of

drunken sailor. The Romans used the plant as an incense and in the Middle Ages the roots were used to perfume linen and clothing. Cats as well as rats are said to be attracted to the plant. In fact this plant is believed to be used by the Pied Piper of Hamelin to lure away the rats from the town. Common valerian has also been used as an aphrodisiac: a girl wearing the plant was said to be never lacking in lovers. English herbalists used to prescribed valerian tea as a strong sedative.

Parts used:
roots: treat spasms, convulsions, hysteria, fever

VERBENA
FAMILY: Verbenaceae
Verbena officinalis 马鞭草
vervain
pigeons' grass
herb of the cross

Verbena is an ancient Latin name of the common European plant, vervain. The Crusaders believed that the plant sprang up at Calvary when the nails were driven into Christ's hands. Vervain thus became commonly known as herb of the cross and was used to sprinkle holy water. Many superstitions are associated with the plant. The Romans regarded it as a plant of good omen. In medieval times

people bathed in water containing the plant in an effort to foresee the future and have their wish come true. The plant was also used as a love potion, to ward off evil spirits, and to prevent dreaming. In A.D. 4, in the court of the Roman emperor Theodosius, vervain was used to treat tumours. The root was cut in half, one half was hung round the patient's neck and the other half placed over a smouldering fire. The tumour was supposed to disappear as the root over the fire shrivelled. This herb, with squarish stem, is cosmopolitan in distribution.

Parts used:
leaves: purgative; increase menstrual flow; induce sweating; expel intestinal worms; antidote for insect bites; quicken expulsion of placenta after birth; treat scurvy, colds, fever, intestinal problems, disorders of the urinary tract, uterine problems

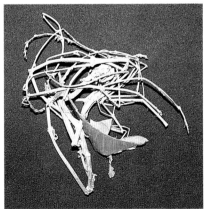

Verbena officinalis

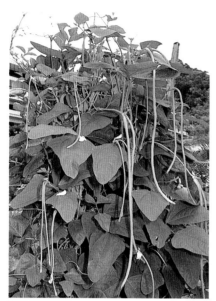

Vigna unguiculata

VIGNA
FAMILY: Leguminosae
Vigna
bean

Vigna is named after Dominicus Vigna, an Italian scientist of the 17th century. These are twining herbs, native from warm temperate to tropical regions of the New World. Characteristics of this group of plants are the leaves, which consist of three leaflets, and the flat pods, which split open to liberate the seeds. Many are grown for the edible seeds and pods.

Vigna angularis 赤豆
adzuki bean
This bean is grown for food in Japan and China.

Parts used:
root: dressing on abscesses

Vigna mungo
black gram
This is widely eaten in India, either boiled as porridge or baked into biscuits and bread. The seeds are considered purgative by the Chinese.

Parts used:
seeds: antidote for vegetable poisoning; treat dysentery, smallpox, urinary problems in old people

Vigna radiata 绿豆
mung bean
This is familiar to many in the form of bean sprouts, which is a popular vegetable.

Parts used:
sprouts: treat threatened abortion

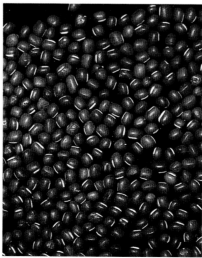

Vigna angularis

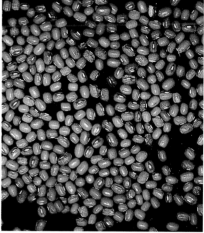

Vigna radiata

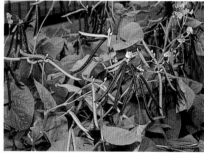

Vigna radiata

Vigna unguiculata subsp. sesquipedalis 长豇豆
asparagus bean
yard-long bean

This plant is native to South Asia. It is characteristic in its metre long, flaccid, or somewhat inflated, pods.

Parts used:
whole plant: quenching and tonic properties; treat diarrhoea, frequent urination
ashes of the pod: induce labour

174

VIOLA
FAMILY: Violaceae
Viola
violets

The generic name of violet, *Viola*, is Latin for "various sweet-smelling flowers". It originates from the Greek *ion*, for "violet", which is named after Io, a daughter of the river god Ianchus. The story behind this is interesting. Jupiter was flirting with Io, and, to conceal this from his wife Juno, changed Io into a heifer. Juno suspected this and asked for the heifer as a gift. So as not to give rise to suspicion, Jupiter consented. Juno then sent the heifer to Argus, a giant with a hundred eyes, to be watched over. Io, who could not run away, grazed on violets. Another Greek legend claimed that violets sprang from the blood of Ajax, a hero of the Trojan War.

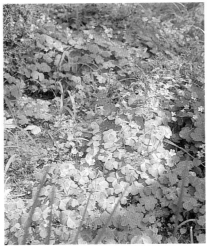
Viola chinensis

Violets are herbs of the temperate regions. In many species, there are two types of flowers – those appearing during early spring are showy and sterile, while those in summer are without petals. Many Asian species of *Viola* are used medicinally by the Chinese.

Viola patrinii 白花地丁
Viola pinnata
whole plant: treats abscesses, cancer

Viola hondoensis
whole plant: treats abscesses

Viola japonica 犁头草
whole plant: wash for inflamed eyes

Viola chinensis
stem: sedative; treats diarrhoea

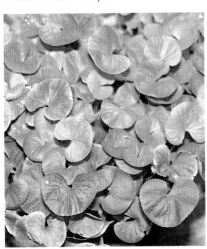
Viola

VITEX
FAMILY: Verbenaceae
Vitex
vitex

These are mostly shrubs and trees, native to tropical and subtropical regions, although a few also occur in temperate areas. The plants have compound leaves, with leaflets arising from the tip of a common stalk.

Vitex negundo 黄荆
Parts used:
seeds: tonic; treat fever; expel phlegm from the respiratory passages
leaves: treat beriberi, headache, chronic dysentery, cholera, dropsy

Vitex trifolia 蔓荆
Parts used:
leaves: contain fever
fruits: treat rheumatism, headache, fever

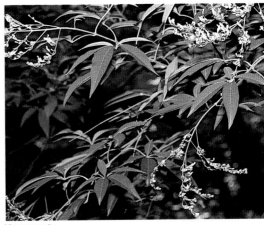
Vitex negundo

175

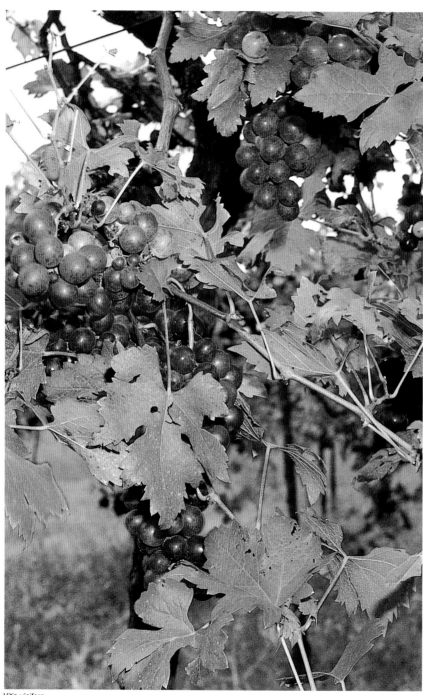

Vitis vinifera

VITIS
FAMILY: Vitaceae
Vitis
grape

Grape plants are woody vines of the northern hemisphere, which climb with the help of tendrils. The generic name *Vitis* is Latin for "vine". The plant is described in some of the oldest ancient writings. In the Bible the plant is frequently mentioned from the time of Noah onwards. In the Christian tradition, grape is an antidote to the fatal apple. It symbolizes the blood of Christ and the Eucharist. The fruits are eaten fresh, or dried as raisins, sultanas and currants, but chiefly made into wine.

Vitis vinifera 葡萄
wine grape
European grape
grape vine
This is the oldest of all cultivated fruits. The cultivation of grape vine was developed into an art by the Greeks and the Romans who introduced the vines and wines to their colonies. Today, wine is an almost universal drink. The plant has been used medicinally by early European herbalists for a number of ailments. The plant sap was used as a lotion for weak eyes and specks on the cornea, and for urinary complaints. The ripe fruits were

used to encourage the flow of urine, to treat smallpox and taken as a tonic. The leaves were used for sore mouths.

Parts used:
roots: induce the secretion of milk in nursing mothers; treat tuberculosis of the lymphatic glands

Vitis thunbergii 蘡薁
Parts used:
sap from the leaves: wash for wounds and swellings

Vitis amurensis 山葡萄
Vitis bryoniaefolia
Vitis flexuosa 葛藟
Parts used:
fruits: tonic

Vitis labrusca
Parts used:
root bark: treats cancerous afflictions

XANTHIUM
FAMILY: Compositae
Xanthium strumarium 苍耳
cocklebur

This is a large branched herb with heart-shaped, hairy leaves. Male and female flowers are borne on separate flowering heads. Fruits are oblong and covered with spines. It is found in wastelands of Japan, Taiwan, China, Korea and Europe and has become naturalized in

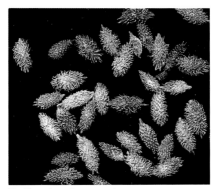
Xanthium strumarium

North America. In southern Europe the leaves, fruits and roots have been used as cures for leprosy, cancer, dysentery and gall bladder problems. Extracts of the plant have been shown to control tumour growth in laboratory animals.

Parts used:
fruits: treat common cold, headache, rheumatic pain, arthritis, inflammation of the nose
stem, leaves: treat German measles

ZANTHOXYLUM
FAMILY: Rutaceae
Zanthoxylum piperitum 秦椒
Japanese prickly ash
Japanese pepper

The generic name, *Zantho-xylum* comes from the Greek words, *xanthos* and *xylon*, meaning "yellow" and "wood". The small tree has brownish,

prickly bark (thus the common name) and paired spines. Flowers are small and yellowish green, with male and female flowers borne on separate trees. Fruits have two valves, each enclosing one shiny black seed. A mountain plant, native to China, Korea, Manchuria and Japan, it is frequently cultivated.

Parts used:
fruits: stimulant; stimulate gastric activities; remove excessive gas in the system; expel intestinal worms
bark: reduces fever
sap of the young leaves: treats insect stings, cat bites

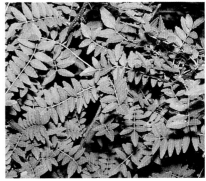
Zanthoxylum piperitum

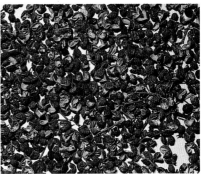
Zanthoxylum piperitum

ZEA

FAMILY: Gramineae

Zea mays 玉蜀黍

maize

corn

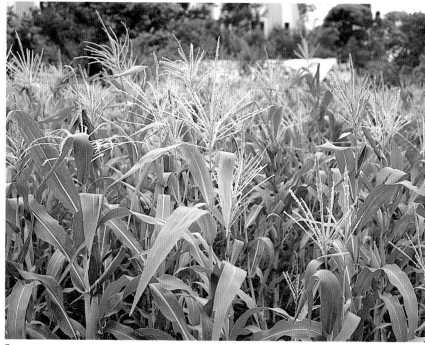
Zea mays

This is a tall herb, with leaves that are arranged in two ranks along the erect, unbranched stem. The stem is jointed, at each joint of which is borne a long, sword-like leaf which curves upwards, then downwards. Male flowers are on long structures growing from the top of the plant. Female flowers grow on a thickened, woody structure, which arises from the axil of the leaves. This structure is wrapped up in many layers of large bracts, at the top of which is a bunch of hairs, known as the tassel or silk. The fruit is the familiar "corn-on-cob". Maize is known only in cultivation. It is of tropical American origin; the wild parent species has long been extinct.

Maize is an important cereal used as a staple, particularly in the tropics, and as a feed for livestock in temperate countries. It is also a raw material for many industrial products such as starch, corn oil, alcohol, acetone and glycerol.

Parts used:

corn silk: stimulant; normalizes flow of urine; soothing effect to the bladder, kidneys and urinary passages when there is inflammation and irritation

empty cob: treats bleeding of the nose and of the uterus

corn hulls: treat diarrhoea in children

roots, leaves: treat urinary difficulties

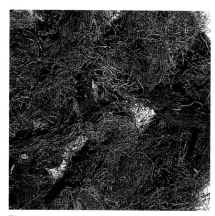
Zea mays

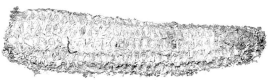
Zea mays

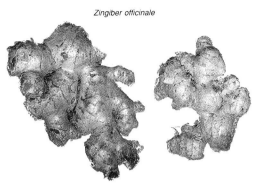

Zingiber officinale

ZINGIBER
FAMILY: Zingiberaceae
Zingiber officinale 姜
ginger

The generic name *Zingiber* comes from Sanskrit. The plant is native to the Pacific islands, but now widely cultivated for its aromatic underground stem, used in cooking. This stem is thick and hard, branched and pale yellow. Arising from the underground stem are tall, erect "stems" made up of closely enveloping leaf sheaths. The yellow flowers are on special stalks arising from the underground stem, one flower from the axil of a flowering bract. Fruits are seldom produced.

   Ginger has been in use as a spice in Asia since ancient times. The underground stem is used variously in cooking: soups, puddings, pickles and curries. Some Chinese cooks keep a piece in the mouth to counter nausea resulting from the fumes of cooking food.

Preserved ginger is an important article of commerce.

Parts used:
underground stem: treats upset stomach, nausea, vomiting, nose bleeds, rheumatism, coughs, blood in stools; improves digestion; expels intestinal gas; stimulates appetite

ZIZIPHUS
FAMILY: Rhamnaceae
Ziziphus jujuba 枣
Chinese jujube
common jujube
Chinese date

Jujubes are known for their fruits, which are preserved dried, pickled or stewed. The spiny plant is native to India and southern China. It grows well in areas which are hot and dry. A large shrub or small tree, often reaching 15 m in height, it bears yellow flowers which develop into reddish-brown fruits. The fruit is elliptical to oblong, and has a dark brown skin covering a whitish pulp which is sweetish.

Parts used:
fruits, seeds: treat anxiety, insomnia, sweating at night, dizziness
bark: treats diarrhoea, fever
roots: treat fever; promote hair growth
leaves: treat scorpion stings

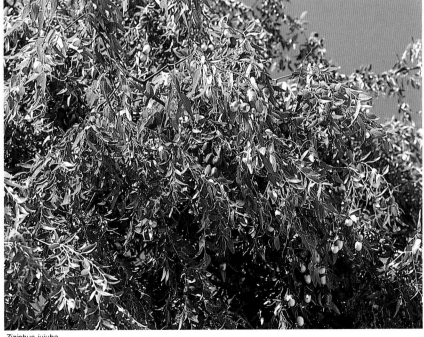

Ziziphus jujuba

INDEX OF COMMON NAMES

INDEX OF CHINESE NAMES （目录）